HOW TO MASTER

NURSING
CALCULATIONS

AUSTRALIAN AND NEW ZEALAND EDITION

HOW TO MASTER

NURSING CALCULATIONS

AUSTRALIAN AND NEW ZEALAND EDITION

Pass numeracy tests and make sense of drug dosage charts

CHRIS TYREMAN
Adapted by PATRICIA FARRAR

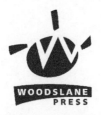

WOODSLANE PRESS

Woodslane Press Pty Ltd
10 Apollo Street
Warriewood, NSW 2102
Email: info@woodslane.com.au
Tel: 02 8445 2300 Website: www.woodslane.com.au

First published in Great Britain in 2008 by Kogan Page Limited
120 Pentonville Road, London N19JN, United Kingdom
This edition published in 2009 in Australia by Woodslane Press
Printed via POD since 2015

A catalogue record for this
book is available from the
National Library of Australia

NATIONAL
LIBRARY
OF AUSTRALIA

Printed in Australia by SOS

Unless you try to do something beyond what you have already mastered, you will never grow.

Ralph Waldo Emerson 1803–1882

Acknowledgments

The publisher would like to acknowledge the contribution of the following reviewers:

Dr Helen Bellchambers Senior Lecturer, School of Nursing and Midwifery, University of Newcastle, NSW.

Jeanette Briscoe RN, BHSc (Nursing), PGDip (Advanced Nursing), CAT, CTT, Senior Nursing Lecturer, NorthTec, NZ.

Ann-Marie Brown Clinical Cordinator, Lecturer in Nursing, Charles Sturt University, Wagga Wagga, NSW.

Clint Douglas RN, PhD, School of Nursing, Queensland University of Technology, QLD.

Robyn Fairhall RN, RM, B.App. Sci (Adv Nsg), MNSt, MRCNA, Monash University, VIC.

Brian Gilchrist BSc, MSc, RN, Director of Nurse Education and Head of School, UCOL, Palmerston North, NZ.

Bronwyn Gordon MN, RN, RM, Paed Cert, School of Nursing, Australian Catholic University, North Sydney, NSW.

Jane Kelly RNcomp, PG Diploma Health Science, School of Nursing, Manukau Institute of Technology, NZ.

Anecita Lim School of Nursing, University of Auckland, NZ.

A/Prof. Violeta Lopez RN, RM, MNA, MPET, PhD, FRCNA, Head of School, School of Nursing, Australian Catholic University, North Sydney, NSW.

Dr Rachel Page Director IFNHH Wellington Campus, Massey University, Wellington, NZ.

Sonia Reisenhofer RN, BN MCN, Undergraduate Campus Student Advisor, Division of Nursing and Midwifery, La Trobe University, Bundoora, VIC.

Vivien Rodgers RN, BA, BN, GDGN, MN, Lecturer, School of Health & Social Sciences, Massey University, Palmerston North, NZ.

Lorraine Walker Lecturer, School of Nursing Gippsland, Monash University, Churchill, VIC.

Contents

Introduction

In health care facilities, most medications are administered by nurses. Consequently it is the nurse who is found responsible for most of the errors made in drug administration. Although errors can occur at any stage in the medication process, from prescription by medical practitioners to delivery to patients by nurses, and in any site in the health care system, it is essential that there are error prevention measures at all levels of medication delivery (Johanna Briggs Institute, 2005).

One source of error is a lack of nursing competence in drug dosage calculations. To promote safe practice, nurse educators can test for poor basic arithmetic skills both at the beginning stage of a program, during the course of education, and at the end of the program. This book teaches the skills necessary for success in these tests at both Enrolled Nurse and Registered Nurse levels. It also explains how to read the medication charts used in the administration of medicines.

The mathematics knowledge required for drug dosage calculation does not exceed lower secondary school standard. You need only the four arithmetic skills of addition (+), subtraction (−), multiplication (×) and division (÷) as applied to whole numbers, fractions and decimal numbers. Tests for student nurses may include medical terms and abbreviations, many of which are obvious, although a few Latin ones need to be remembered.

The book caters for most levels of mathematical ability, so it is suitable for mature students who have had little experience of numerical work since leaving school. Even candidates with very poor numerical skills should find it helpful. Because calculators are not usually allowed in an examination room, it is vital that you can understand basic arithmetic processes and solve problems 'in you head' using mental arithmetic or by writing the calculation on paper.

The first two chapters will familiarise you with the key topics of arithmetic, fractions, decimals and percentages. Chapter 3 introduces the metric system of measurement as appropriate to nursing. Chapter 4 covers drug dosage calculations, starting with simple problems that require only one or two arithmetic steps before moving on to more complicated calculations that require several arithmetic steps. Chapter 5 covers drug names and medication charts, or treatment sheets, as they are known. It tests your ability to administer the right drug in the right amount to the right patient via the right route at the right time – the five Rs of drug administration. It is not intended to test your knowledge of drugs, only your ability to read charts and carry out simple mathematical calculations. In practice you will need to reflect on normal doses, the purpose of the medication (its indication), unwanted side effects and adverse reactions. These skills are essential for the safe administration of medications but are not part of this book.

You are advised to work systematically through the book from start to finish, completing the in-text questions. The answers are to be found at the end of the book. If any chapter is too simple or does meet your learning needs, then skip to the questions at the end of the chapter. If you can answer all of the questions correctly, you already have the essential knowledge for safe drug calculation and can move on to the next chapter.

The final chapter of the book contains practice questions of the type usually found in medication calculation tests. A basic numerical test is followed by three nursing calculation mock tests of 50 questions each. You have one hour to complete each of the mock tests and the pass mark is 100 per cent. You are advised to repeat those items that you did not answer correctly and to note where you made mistakes. Errors in drug administration are unacceptable and always require further investigation. When you are out on the wards the pass mark is always 100 per cent!

Reference

Johanna Briggs Institute (2005). Strategies to reduce medication errors with reference to older adults. *Best Practice (9)*, 4, p 1-6.

The following sources have been used to cross-check drug names and dosages in current use in Australia and New Zealand:

Australian Medicines Handbook. http:www.amh.net.au

Lim, A.G. (Ed.) (2008). *Australia New Zealand Nursing & Midwifery Drug Handbook (4th ed.)* Broadway, NSW: Lippincott Williams & Wilkins.

MIMS Online. http://www.mims.com.au

Society of Hospital Pharmacists Australia. (2008). http://www.shpa.org.au

Tiziani, A. (2004). *Havard's Nursing Guide to Drugs (7th ed.)*. Sydney: Elsevier

Basic maths self-assessment test

Nursing students come from varied backgrounds and have different employment and education experiences. The following test is aimed at students making a fresh start in education. It will reveal any gaps in your mathematical knowledge. There are three levels of difficulty: revision, level 1 and level 2, with 10 questions at each level. If you make any mistakes at the remedial level, you may have a particular problem that is beyond the scope of this book and you are advised to seek assistance. However, you should study the first eight pages of Chapter 1 and attempt the first two exercises before seeking help.

Students should be able to answer all of the questions at level 1 correctly. Wrong answers at this stage can be rectified by studying the first three chapters. Success at level 2 requires a firm foundation in numeracy. Mistakes made at this level will help you to identify those topics that need particular attention: for example, fractions, decimals, percentages or the metric system. Competency in these skills is essential for drug dosage calculations.

The test has no time limit nor does it require any knowledge of drug administration; calculators are not allowed. Answers can be found at the end of the book. There is no 'pass' mark but you can check your results against the following guide to numerical competency:

- Fewer than 10 correct answers: you may have numerical difficulties that require help.
- 10 to 14 marks: you can recognise numbers and count but have problems with simple arithmetic problems.
- 15 to 20 marks: you have a grasp of basic arithmetic but have little knowledge of fractions, decimals or percentages.
- 21 to 25 marks: you have competent number skills but these could be extended further.
- 26 to 30 marks: you possess most of the basic skills necessary for success in drug dosage calculations.

Revision

1. Write out 25 in words.
2. Write out 4060 in words.
3. Write out 980 107 in words.
4. Write out three thousand and thirty in figures.
5. Write out one million two hundred and ten thousand in figures.
6. Here are two numbers: 4900 and 12 500. Which is the larger?
7. Here are two numbers: 0.3 and 0.09. Which is the larger?

8. What does the 2 mean in 7250?
9. How many cents is $0.75?
10. If it is 8.30 pm now, what time will it be in 3 hours?

Level 1

11. 7 + 9 + 4 =
12. 957 + 63 =
13. 212 − 76 =
14. 32 × 9 =
15. 315 ÷ 5 =
16. How many more than 27 is 42?
17. What change should be handed over when a bill of $16.23 is paid with a $20 note?
18. Overnight the temperature rose from −1 °C to + 4 °C. By how many degrees did it rise?
19. On average, a salesperson drives 720 km per week. How many kilometres are driven per annum?
20. A lottery syndicate wins $225,000. If there are 20 people in the syndicate, how much will each person receive?

Level 2

21. $5\frac{1}{2} + 2\frac{1}{4} =$
22. $1\frac{2}{3} \div \frac{5}{9} =$
23. 8.2 + 7.45 =
24. 4.5 × 6 =
25. 38 ÷ 0.5 =
26. Find the interest paid on $8500 borrowed for 1 year at an interest rate of 12 per cent per annum.
27. Write 20% as a fraction.
28. Write 45% as a decimal.
29. How many milligrams are there in 0.25 grams?
30. Write 1.455 corrected to two decimal places.

1 Basic arithmetic skills

How to add, subtract, multiply and divide whole numbers

This first chapter is a refresher course in the basic arithmetic skills required for any mathematics test. If you find it too easy you can skip directly to the end-of-chapter questions. However, if you get any of the answers wrong you may have a numeracy problem that requires remedial help.

Numbers and place value

Starting at the simplest level, our number system is easily understood if you consider 'place value' where each number from 0 to 9 is written in a column – units, tens, hundreds and so on.

Numbers in words	Numbers in figures			
	Thou.	Hun.	Tens	Units
one hundred and seven	–	1	0	7
seven thousand two hundred	7	2	0	0
twenty five	–	–	2	5

Addition

Numbers to be added must be arranged underneath each other so that the unit columns are in line.

Example: 139 + 226

The first step is to align the numbers in columns.

$$
\begin{array}{c|c|c}
1 & 3 & 9 \\
2 & 2 & 6 +
\end{array}
$$

Then we add the units column (right-hand column) 6 + 9 = 15.

The 5 is placed in the units column and the 10 carried over as one 'ten' into the tens column.

$$
\begin{array}{r}
1\ 3\ 9 \\
2\ 2\ 6\ + \\
\hline
5 \\
\hline
1
\end{array}
$$

Now we add the tens column (middle column) remembering to include the 1 that has been carried:

1 + 2 + 3 = 6 (middle column):

$$
\begin{array}{r}
1\ 3\ 9 \\
2\ 2\ 6\ + \\
\hline
6\ 5 \\
\hline
1
\end{array}
$$

Now we add the hundreds column: 2 + 1 = 3 (left-hand column).

$$
\begin{array}{r}
1\ 3\ 9 \\
2\ 2\ 6\ + \\
\hline
3\ 6\ 5 \\
\hline
1
\end{array}
$$

For the addition of three or more numbers, the method is the same.

Example: 200 + 86 + 44 becomes:

```
  2 0 0
    8 6 +
    4 4
  3 3 0
  1 1
```

Subtraction

Subtraction is concerned with taking things away. Subtraction is the reverse of addition. The most important thing about subtraction is that the larger number is on top (above the smaller), so when subtracting numbers you *subtract the smaller number from the bigger number.*

As with addition, the numbers must be arranged underneath each other, so that the units columns are in line. After aligning the numbers, we subtract (take away) the columns vertically, starting at the right-hand end (units column).

For example: 374 − 126

```
  3 7 4
  1 2 6 −
```

The first step is to align the numbers:

The next step is to subtract the units column (the right-hand column): but 4 − 6 we cannot do since 6 is larger than 4. To overcome this problem we borrow 1 from the tens column (this is the same as 10 units) and add it to the 4 in the units column. So our sum now becomes:

14 − 6 (which we can do) = 8

So far we can write:

```
  3 7 4
  1 2 6 −
      8
```

The next step is to pay back the '1' we have just borrowed from the tens column. There are two methods for doing this and both are now explained.

Method 1 (old-fashioned method – most popular)
In this method the 10 is paid back to the bottom, for example:

$$
\begin{array}{r}
3\ 7\ ^{1}4 \\
1\ 2_{1}6\ - \\
\hline
8
\end{array}
$$

Now we add the 1 and the 2 to make 3. The 3 is subtracted from the 7 to give to the 4. So the sum becomes:

$$
\begin{array}{r}
3\ 7\ ^{1}4 \\
1\ 2_{1}6\ - \\
\hline
4\ 8
\end{array}
$$

Finally we subtract the 1 from 3 (in the hundreds column) to give 2:

$$
\begin{array}{r}
3\ 7\ ^{1}4 \\
1\ 2_{1}6\ - \\
\hline
2\ 4\ 8
\end{array}
$$

Method 2 (modern method)
In this method the 10 borrowed is subtracted as a 1 at the top of the tens column (7 – 1 = 6), so:

$$
\begin{array}{r}
3\ 7^{6}\ ^{1}4 \\
1\ 2_{1}\ \ 6\ - \\
\hline
2\ 4\ \ 8
\end{array}
$$

Now try the following questions. *You must not use a calculator* for any questions in this book. Try to work out the answer 'in your head' if possible, otherwise do your working out on a separate sheet of paper.

Test 1

Write out the following numbers in figures:

1. one thousand one hundred and sixty eight.
2. nine thousand and forty two.
3. two thousand and nine.
4. twenty seven thousand five hundred and fifty.

Work out the following additions and subtractions:

5. $409 + 24 =$
6. $250 + 17\ 800 =$
7. $1427 - 300 =$
8. $6742 - 5630 =$

If any of your answers are wrong in Test 1 you may have a numeracy problem that requires remedial help.

Multiplication

Multiplication (or 'times') means 'lots of', and is a quick way of adding up numbers that have an equal value.

For example: 5 multiplied by 3 = 5 + 5 + 5.

Note that $5 \times 3 = 15$ and $3 \times 5 = 15$.

This applies to all numbers that are multiplied together: it does not matter which way around you put them, the answer is the same.

To work with multiplication sums you must be familiar with your 'times tables'. The most common times tables are shown in Table 1.2.

The multiplication table in Table 1.1 is a handy way of finding the answer (known as the 'product') when any two numbers from 1 to 12 are multiplied together. See whether you can find out how to use it – it's not difficult!

Short multiplication

This is the term for the multiplication of any number by a unit (1 to 9).

Table 1.1 Multiplication table (try to memorise it)

	1	2	3	4	5	6	7	8	9	10	11	12
1	1	2	3	4	5	6	7	8	9	10	11	12
2	2	4	6	8	10	12	14	16	18	21	22	24
3	3	6	9	12	15	18	21	24	27	30	33	36
4	4	8	12	16	20	24	28	32	36	40	44	48
5	5	10	15	20	25	30	35	40	45	50	55	60
6	6	12	18	24	30	36	42	48	54	60	66	72
7	7	14	21	28	35	42	49	56	63	70	77	84
8	8	16	24	32	40	48	56	64	72	80	88	96
9	9	18	27	36	45	54	63	72	81	90	99	108
10	10	20	30	40	50	60	70	80	90	100	110	120
11	11	22	33	44	55	66	77	88	99	110	121	132
12	12	24	36	48	60	72	84	96	108	120	132	144

Examples are:

$$3 \times 8$$
$$3\,2 \times 4$$
$$1\,0\,8 \times 9$$
$$5\,2\,4 \times 3$$
↑ All units

For example: 19 × 3. We write the sum as:

$$1\,9$$
$$3 \times$$

First we multiply the 9 by the 3 to give 27:

9 × 3 = 27 (see three times table).

As with addition the 7 is written in the units column and the 2 is carried as two tens into the tens column as follows:

$$\begin{array}{r} 1\,9 \\ 3\,\times \\ \hline 7 \\ {}_{2} \end{array}$$

Table 1.2 The common times tables

2 times	3 times	4 times	5 times	6 times	7 times
1×2 = 2	1×3 = 3	1×4 = 4	1×5 = 5	1×6 = 6	1×7 = 7
2×2 = 4	2×3 = 6	2×4 = 8	2×5 = 10	2×6 = 12	2×7 = 14
3×2 = 6	3×3 = 9	3×4 = 12	3×5 = 15	3×6 = 18	3×7 = 21
4×2 = 8	4×3 = 12	4×4 = 16	4×5 = 20	4×6 = 24	4×7 = 28
5×2 = 10	5×3 = 15	5×4 = 20	5×5 = 25	5×6 = 30	5×7 = 35
6×2 = 12	6×3 = 18	6×4 = 24	6×5 = 30	6×6 = 36	6×7 = 42
7×2 = 14	7×3 = 21	7×4 = 28	7×5 = 35	7×6 = 42	7×7 = 49
8×2 = 16	8×3 = 24	8×4 = 32	8×5 = 40	8×6 = 48	8×7 = 56
9×2 = 18	9×3 = 27	9×4 = 36	9×5 = 45	9×6 = 54	9×7 = 63
0×2 = 20	10×3 = 30	10×4 = 40	10×5 = 50	10×6 = 60	10×7 = 70
11×2 = 22	11×3 = 33	11×4 = 44	11×5 = 55	11×6 = 66	11×7 = 77
12×2 = 24	12×3 = 36	12×4 = 48	12×5 = 60	12×6 = 72	12×7 = 84

8 times	9 times	10 times	11 times	12 times
1×8 = 8	1×9 = 9	1×10 = 10	1×11 = 11	1×12 = 12
2×8 = 16	2×9 = 18	2×10 = 20	2×11 = 22	2×12 = 24
3×8 = 24	3×9 = 27	3×10 = 30	3×11 = 33	3×12 = 36
4×8 = 32	4×9 = 36	4×10 = 40	4×11 = 44	4×12 = 48
5×8 = 40	5×9 = 45	5×10 = 50	5×11 = 55	5×12 = 60
6×8 = 48	6×9 = 54	6×10 = 60	6×11 = 66	6×12 = 72
7×8 = 56	7×9 = 63	7×10 = 70	7×11 = 77	7×12 = 84
8×8 = 64	8×9 = 72	8×10 = 80	8×11 = 88	8×12 = 96
9×8 = 72	9×9 = 81	9×10 = 90	9×11 = 99	9×12 = 108
10×8 = 80	10×9 = 90	10×10 = 100	10×11 = 110	10×12 = 120
11×8 = 88	11×9 = 99	11×10 = 110	11×11 = 121	11×12 = 132
12×8 = 96	12×9 = 108	12×10 = 120	12×11 = 132	12×12 = 144

Now we multiply the 1 by the 3 to give 3 ($1 \times 3 = 3$). This 3 is added to the 2 previously carried to the tens column to give 5, so the finished sum becomes:

$$
\begin{array}{r}
1\,9 \\
3\times \\
\hline
5\,7 \\
\scriptstyle 2
\end{array}
$$

so $19 \times 3 = 57$.

Example: what is 68 × 9? We rewrite the sum as:

$$6\,8$$
$$9 \times$$

Multiplying the units gives 8 × 9 = 72 (see nine times table), so we have:

$$6\,8$$
$$\underline{9 \times}$$
$$\underline{2}$$
$$\small 7$$

We multiply the 6 in the tens column by the 9 to give 6 × 9 = 54. The 54 is added to the 7 previously carried, to give 54 + 7 = 61. The 1 of the 61 is placed in the tens column and the 6 of the 61 is carried into the hundreds column:

$$6\,8$$
$$\underline{9 \times}$$
$$\underline{1\,2}$$
$$\small 6\,7$$

Since there are no hundreds to multiply in the hundreds column, the figure 6 can be carried directly into this column, giving:

$$6\,8$$
$$\underline{9 \times}$$
$$\underline{6\,1\,2}$$
$$\small 6\,7$$

Test 2

Calculate the following multiplication sums:
1. 7 × 9
2. 12 × 8
3. Multiply 20 by 6.
4. Multiply 23 by 4.
5. 90 times 5 is …
6. The product of 19 and 5 is …
7. 33 × 3

8. 75×4
9. 125×8
10. 11×12

Long multiplication

This is the term for multiplying any number by a number greater than 9, for example 52×18 or 120×50.

To multiply 52×18 we rewrite this as:

$$
\begin{array}{r}
5\,2 \\
1\,8\,\times \\
\hline
\end{array}
$$

We proceed in two steps as follows. First we multiply the 52 by the 8 in the units column and second we multiply the 52 by the 1 in the tens column.

First step: (multiply 52 by the 8) so we have:

$$
\begin{array}{r}
5\,2 \\
1\,8\,\times \\
\hline
4\,1\,6 \\
\scriptstyle 1
\end{array}
$$

Second step (multiply the 52 by the 1 in the tens column). Since we are now multiplying from the tens column we leave the units column blank, which is the same as filling it with a 0. The sum is written on the line below 416:

$$
\begin{array}{r}
5\,2 \\
1\,8\,\times \\
\hline
4\,1\,6 \\
5\,2\,0
\end{array}
$$

We now add the two steps together: add 416 and 520 to give the final sum which is shown below:

$$
\begin{array}{r}
5\,2 \\
1\,8\,\times \\
\hline
4\,1\,6 \\
5\,2\,0 \\
\hline
9\,3\,6
\end{array}
$$

Test 3

Work out the following multiplication sums:

1. 62×13 6. 125×80
2. 79×32 7. 167×33
3. 80×15 8. 42×121
4. 254×20 9. 195×205
5. 17×25 10. 13×54

Division

Division is the reverse of multiplication, and is concerned with sharing (or dividing numbers into equal parts).

Example: divide 195 by 3. So we have $195 \div 3$ which is rewritten

$$3\overline{\smash{)}1\ 9\ 5}$$

The first step is to divide the 1 by the 3. However, since 3 into 1 won't go, we have to carry the 1 into the next column, so:

$$3\overline{\smash{)}1\ ^{1}9\ 5}$$

We now use the multiplication table in reverse to find how many 3s are in 19. To do this start in the 3s column on the left-hand side and move along the horizontal row until you get to the number that is closest to but smaller than 19. The number is 18. Following the vertical row upwards gives us 6. So 3 goes into 19 six times with 1 left over ($19 - 18 = 1$ left over). The 6 is placed at the top; the 1 is carried to the next column to make 15.

$$3\overline{\smash{)}1\ ^{1}9\ ^{1}5}^{\,6}$$

Finally the 3 is divided into 15. The three times table shows us that 3 goes into 15 times exactly, so the finished sum is:

$$3\overline{\smash{)}1\ ^{1}9\ ^{1}5}^{\,6\ 5}$$

The answer can be checked by multiplying it by the number that we have divided by (65 × 3 = 195: correct).

Test 4

Work out the following divisions:
1. 36 ÷ 9   5. 1230 ÷ 3
2. 248 ÷ 4   6. 295 ÷ 5
3. 3⟌339   7. 1464 ÷ 6
4. 5⟌265   8. 1000 ÷ 8

Long division
This is the term for division by large numbers.

Example: for 2064 divided by 48 we write: 48⟌2064
First step: divide 2 by 48 – won't go
Second step: divide 20 by 48 – won't go
Third step: divide 206 by 48 – will go
48 into 206 will go, but we don't have a times table for 48 so we have to *build up a table ourselves*. This is done as follows:

1 × 48 = 48
2 × 48 = 96
3 × 48 = 144
4 × 48 = 192 (the nearest to 206)
5 × 48 = 240 (too big)

Fourth step: work out the remainder. We know that 48 goes into 206 four times to leave a remainder of 14 (206 – 192 = 14).

```
            4
   4 8│2 0 6 4
       │1 9 2 -
          1 4
```

Fifth step: we now bring the 4 down to give 144:

```
            4
   4 8│2 0 6 4
       │1 9 2 -
          1 4 4
```

Sixth step: the 48 is divided into 144 to give 3 with no remainder (see 48 times table on page xxs).

```
              4 3
    4 8 | 2 0 6 4
          1 9 2 -
            1 4 4
            1 4 4 -
```

So, 2064 ÷ 48 = 43.

Test 5

Work out the following long division sums:
1. 360 ÷ 12   6. 216 ÷ 36
2. 372 ÷ 12   7. 950 ÷ 25
3. 18⟌792   8. 2680 ÷ 40
4. 20⟌900   9. 976 ÷ 16
5. 72⟌1440   10. 4944 ÷ 24

By now you should be familiar with the four basic rules of arithmetic: that is, how to add, subtract, multiply and divide whole numbers. The next chapter explains how to use these maths skills with fractions and decimals.

Sequence of operations ('BoDMAS')

A calculation with two or more arithmetic signs (or operations) must be worked out in the correct sequence, which is:

Division and multiplication before addition and subtraction.

You can remember the sequence of operations as **BoDMAS**: **B**rackets, **D**ivision, **M**ultiplication, **A**ddition and **S**ubtraction.

Example: $4 \times 3 + 6$

Multiplication first: $4 \times 3 = 12$ followed by addition: $12 + 6 = 18$

So $4 \times 3 + 6 = 18$

If we carried out the addition part first $(3 + 6 = 9)$ and then multiplied by the 4 this would have given 36 $(4 \times 9 = 36)$, which is the wrong answer.

Example: $25 - 12 \div 3$

Division first: $12 \div 3 = 4$ followed by subtraction $25 - 4 = 21$

So $25 - 12 \div 3 = 21$

Where a calculation contains only addition and subtraction, each part is worked out in a sequence from left to right.

Example: $11 - 3 + 9 - 2$ becomes $11 - 3 = 8$ then $8 + 9 = 17$ then finally $17 - 2 = 15$

Where a calculation contains only multiplication and division, each part out is worked out in sequence from left to right.

Example: $10 \div 2 \times 6$ becomes $10 \div 2 = 5$ followed by $5 \times 6 = 30$

Test 6

Work out the following (without using a calculator):

1. $12 \div 6 + 12$
2. $10 + 15 \div 5$
3. $3 \times 4 - 2$
4. $8 - 3 \times 2$
5. $10 + 20 \div 5$
6. $15 - 9 + 3$
7. $14 + 11 - 10 - 6 =$
8. $22 \times 4 \div 2 + 12 =$
9. $30 \div 6 \times 5 - 15 =$
10. $2 \times 3 \times 4 \times 5 \div 20 =$
11. $10 - 1 \times 3 - 1 =$
12. $9 + 3 \times 4 \div 2 - 1 =$

Some calculations include brackets to help make sure that the arithmetic is carried out in the correct sequence. Where a calculation contains brackets, the sum inside the brackets must be worked out first.

Example: $12 \div (6 - 2)$
First step: $(6 - 2) = 4$
Second step $12 \div 4 = 3$
So $12 \div (6 - 2) = 3$

Without the brackets, $12 \div 6 - 2$ is $12 \div 6 = 2$, then $2 - 2 = 0$.

Finally, you should be aware that when no arithmetic sign is placed outside the brackets, the calculation is automatically taken as being times ($\times$). This rule applies to every calculation where there is no sign outside the bracket. So $9(6 + 5)$ means $9 \times (6 + 5)$ and the sum becomes $9 \times 11 = 99$.

Test 7

Calculate the following by working out the brackets first:

1.	$9 + (5 \times 3)$	7.	$3(10 + 6 \div 2)$
2.	$14 - (10 + 2)$	8.	$3 + 6(4 \times 2 + 1)$
3.	$30 \div (3 \times 2)$	9.	$2(23 - 17) \div 4$
4.	$4 \times (20 - 9)$	10.	$4 + 4(4 + 4)$
5.	$10(10 - 9)$	11.	$90 \div 9(8 - 3 \times 2)$
6.	$7 (15 \div 5)$	12.	$10 \times 2(60 \div 2 \times 15)$

Factors and multiples

Skill with numbers will help you to work out drug dosage calculations without having to use a calculator. The ability to break down large numbers is an essential part of working with fractions. The latter form the basis of many drug calculations.

Factors are numbers that will divide into another number exactly, without leaving a remainder. For example:

15 is a factor of 60 (60 divided by 15 = 4)
50 is a factor of 250 (250 divided by 50 = 5)
100 is a factor of 1000 (1000 divided by 100 = 10)

All the factors of a number are all of the whole numbers that will divide into it exactly. Take the number 36 for example. The factors of 36 are:

1 and 36
2 and 18
3 and 12
4 and 9
6 and 6

Notice how the factors are found in pairs. Pairing off in this way will help you to find the factors of large numbers, without missing any out. The factors of 36 can be listed as:

1 2 3 4 6 9 12 18 and 36.

The highest common factor (HCF) of two numbers is the highest of their common factors. For example: what is the highest common factor of 60 and 15?

15: factors = 1 3 5 15
60: factors = 1 2 3 4 5 6 10 12 15 20 30 60

The factors that are common to both 15 and 60 are 1, 3, 5 and 15, and of these 15 is the highest, so 15 is the HCF of 60 and 15. Example: what is the HCF of 20 and 16?

16: 1 2 4 8 16

20: 1 2 4 5 10 20

1, 2 and 4 are the common factors so 4 is the HCF of 16 and 20.

Test 8

Find the factors of the following numbers. Use the pairing-off method (1 and; 2 and; 3 and; 4 and; 5 and; 6 and; etc):
1. 6 (four factors)
2. 10 (four factors)
3. 32 (six factors)
4. 90 (12 factors)
5. 500 (12 factors)

Find the highest common factor (HCF) of:
6. 24 and 32
7. 75 and 120
8. 12 and 500
9. 50 and 1000
10. 25 and 400

A *prime number* is a number that is only divisible by itself and 1. It has only two factors – the number itself and 1. The lowest prime number is 2 (1 is not a prime number because it has only one factor – itself).

All the prime numbers below 50 are listed below:

2 3 5 7 11 13 17 19 23 29 31 37 41 43 47

Note: with the exception of 2 all the prime numbers are odd numbers (but not all odd numbers are prime numbers).

A factor that is a prime number is called a *prime factor*. To find the prime factors of any number we keep dividing by prime numbers – starting with the lowest prime number that will divide into it, and then progressing through until it will not divide by any prime number any further.

Example: what are the prime factors of 210?

$210 \div 2 = 105$
$105 \div 3 = 35$
$35 \div 5 = 7$
$7 \div 7 = 1$

So 210 has the prime factors 2, 3, 5, and 7.

$210 = 2 \times 3 \times 5 \times 7$

Example: express 2520 as a product of its prime factors.
As in the previous example we start dividing by the lowest prime number, which is 2:

$2520 \div 2 = 1260$

1260 is an even number so it will divide by 2 again:

$1260 \div 2 = 630$

630 is an even number so it will divide by 2 again:

$630 \div 2 = 315$

315 is an odd number so it will not divide by 2 but it will divide by the next prime number which is 3:

$315 \div 3 = 105$

105 will divide by 3 again:

$105 \div 3 = 35$

35 will not divide by 3, but it will divide by the next prime number which is 5:

$35 \div 5 = 7$

7 is a prime number so it will not divide any further.

$7 \div 7 = 1$

So, $2520 = 2 \times 2 \times 2 \times 3 \times 3 \times 5 \times 7$.

Note: finding the correct prime factors involves trial and error if the number does not divide by the first prime factor you try.
$209 \div 2 = 104$ remainder 1, so 2 is not a prime factor of 209.
$209 \div 3 = 69$ remainder 2, so 3 is not a prime factor of 209.
$209 \div 5 = 41$ remainder 4, so 5 is not a prime factor of 209.
$209 \div 7 = 29$ remainder 6, so 7 is not a prime factor of 209.
$209 \div 11 = 19$ exactly so 11 is a prime factor of 209.

From this we can see that 209 has the prime factors 11 and 19.

Test 9

Express the following numbers as a product of their prime factors
(2 3 5 7 11 13, etc.):

1.	6	5.	81
2.	30	6.	216
3.	63	7.	125
4.	420	8.	343

A *multiple* of a number is the number multiplied by:

1 2 3 4 5 6 7 8 9 10 11 12 13 14, etc.

So a multiple is the 'times table' of a number. For example:

The multiples of 5 are: 5 10 15 20 25 30, etc.

The multiples of 6 are: 6 12 18 24 30, etc.

The multiples of 10 are: 10 20 30 40 50, etc.

Common multiples are those numbers that are common to a pair
of numbers. For example, what are the first three common
multiples of 5 and 10?

multiples of 5: 5 <u>10</u> 15 <u>20</u> 25 <u>30</u>

multiples of 10: <u>10</u> <u>20</u> <u>30</u> 40 50

The common numbers are underlined, so the first three common
multiples of 5 and 10 are: 10, 20 and 30. The lowest of these is 10,
making it the lowest common multiple (LCM); it is the lowest
number that both 5 and 10 will divide into exactly.

Example: Find the lowest common multiple (LCM) of 3 and 9.

multiples of 3: 3 6 9 12 18
multiples of 9: 9 18 27 36 45
so the LCM of 3 and 9 is 9.

Example: Find the lowest common multiple (LCM) of 4 and 5.
4: 4 8 12 16 20 24
5: 5 10 15 20 25
so LCM is 20.

Test 10

Find the first four multiples of:
1. 2
2. 12
3. 20
4. 25
5. 100

Find the lowest common multiple (LCM) of:
6. 2 and 3
7. 12 and 20
8. 24 and 36
9. 30 and 75
10. 25 and 40

Chapter 1 questions

1. Write out two thousand and twenty two in figures.
2. Add 434 and 176.
3. Subtract 51 from 246.
4. Subtract 2750 from 5342.
5. Multiply 9 by 12.
6. Multiply 8 × 8.
7. Multiply 125 × 45.
8. Multiply 1053 × 141.
9. Divide 121 by 11.
10. Divide 195 by 5.
11. Divide 3136 by 14.
12. Divide 1728 by 24.
13. Divide 1040 by 8.
14. $10 + 20 \div 2 =$
15. $20 \div 2 \times 10 =$
16. $10 + 4 - 5 + 7 =$
17. $8 \times 3 \div 4 \times 9 =$
18. $10(5 + 3) =$
19. $2(8 + 10 \div 2) =$

20. $3 \times 5(12 \div 3 + 6) =$
21. Find the factors of 20.
22. What are the prime factors of 20?
23. Find the factors of 42.
24. What are the prime factors of 42?
25. Write down the first six multiples of 6.
26. Write down the first six multiples of 9.
27. What is the lowest common multiple of 6 and 9?
28. What is the lowest common multiple of 20 and 25?
29. What is the lowest common multiple of 50 and 250?
30. What is the lowest common multiple of 10 and 12?

2 Fractions and decimals

Introduction to fractions

We use fractions in everyday situations; for example, we talk about *half* an hour, *three-quarters* of a cup or shops selling goods with a discount of *one-third*.

½ hour ¾ cup ⅓ discount

You will be familiar with these everyday examples of fractions. Each of these fractions consists of part of the whole, so they indicate part of an hour, part of a cup and part of the price.

So a fraction is: the whole divided into a number of equal parts.

All fractions have a top and bottom number. The bottom number, or *denominator*, tells us how many equal parts the whole is divided into. The top number, or *numerator*, tells us how many parts we have. So half an hour means that we divide the hour into two equal parts and we have one part.

An easy way to understand fractions is to draw the whole in diagram form and shade in the fraction. For example:

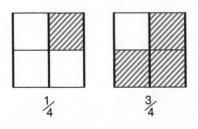

Cancelling (equivalent fractions)

Some fractions can be cancelled so as to express them in smaller numbers. The value of the fraction is not altered by cancelling and so the outcome is an *equivalent fraction*.

For example, four-sixths can be expressed as a fraction having smaller numbers, by dividing both the top and bottom numbers by 2. This is known as cancelling.

$$\frac{4}{6}\begin{smallmatrix}\div2\\\div2\end{smallmatrix}=\frac{2}{3}$$

Remember, the value of the fraction has not become smaller, only the numbers involved – this means that *four-sixths* and *two-thirds* are equivalent fractions:

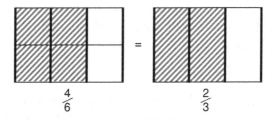

Another example of cancelling is $^8/_{16}$. This fraction can be cancelled three times as follows:

$^8/_{16}$ can be cancelled to $^4/_8$ by dividing the 8 and the 16 by 2.
$^8/_{16}$ can be cancelled to $^2/_4$ by dividing the 8 and the 16 by 4.
$^8/_{16}$ can be cancelled to $^1/_2$ by dividing the 8 and the 16 by 8.

So the equivalent fractions are $^8/_{16} = ^4/_8 = ^2/_4 = ^1/_2$.

If we cancel $^8/_{16}$ to $^1/_2$ this is known as cancelling a fraction to its lowest terms (it cannot be reduced any further).

Test 11

Cancel the following fractions to their lowest terms (hints given):

1. $^3/_6$ (divide the top and the bottom by 3).
2. $^{15}/_{20}$ (divide the top and the bottom by 5).
3. $^{12}/_{36}$ (divide the top and bottom by 12, or by 2, 2, and 3).
4. $^{40}/_{72}$ (divide by the smallest prime number, three times over).
5. $^{16}/_{24}$ (try dividing by small prime numbers).
6. $^{18}/_{30}$ (try dividing by small prime numbers).
7. $^{10}/_{100}$ (numbers ending in zero always divide by 10).
8. $^{95}/_{100}$ (numbers ending in 5 always divide by 5).
9. $^8/_{12}$ (use the methods outlined above).
10. $^{40}/_{100}$ (use the methods outlined above).

How to add and subtract fractions

Addition and subtraction of fractions can be dealt with together as the same 'rules' apply to both. Multiplication and division of fractions have different rules and will be explained separately.

For us to be able to add or subtract fractions they must have the same denominators. Take the following example:

$$\frac{1}{8} + \frac{3}{8}$$

Both fractions have a denominator of 8. We write the denominator *once*, and then add the two top numbers:

$$\text{so } \frac{1}{8} + \frac{3}{8} = \frac{1+3}{8} = \frac{4}{8}$$

An example of subtraction is:

$$\frac{13}{16} - \frac{5}{16} = \frac{13-5}{16} = \frac{8}{16}$$

Test 12

Add/subtract the following fractions then cancel where possible (questions 5 to 8):

1. $\frac{6}{8} + \frac{1}{8}$ 5. $\frac{7}{9} - \frac{2}{9} + \frac{4}{9}$
2. $\frac{2}{6} + \frac{3}{6}$ 6. $\frac{11}{12} - \frac{5}{12}$
3. $\frac{7}{10} - \frac{4}{10}$ 7. $\frac{9}{15} + \frac{1}{15}$
4. $\frac{11}{12} - \frac{4}{12}$ 8. $\frac{12}{40} + \frac{4}{40}$

When the fractions have different denominators we can still add or subtract them, but in order to do so we first of all have to find a *common denominator*. This is a number that both denominators will divide into. Take the following example:

$$\frac{1}{4} + \frac{3}{6}$$

The first fraction has a denominator of 4 and the second fraction has a denominator of 6. The *common denominator* is a number that both 4 and 6 will divide into. There are many numbers that both 4 and 6 will divide into. To find them we compare the 4 times table with the 6 times table and see where they give us the same answer. From these tables, we can see that 4 and 6 have common denominators at 12, 24, 36 and 48. To make the working easier we choose the lowest of these, 12 (the lowest common factor as explained in Chapter 1).

4 times	6 times
1×4 = 4	1×6 = 6
2×4 = 8	2×6 = **12**
3×4 = **12**	3×6 = 18
4×4 = 16	4×6 = **24**
5×4 = 20	5×6 = 30
6×4 = **24**	6×6 = **36**
7×4 = 28	7×6 = 42
8×4 = 32	8×6 = **48**
9×4 = **36**	9×6 = 54
10×4 = 40	10×6 = 60
11×4 = 44	11×6 = 66
12×4 = **48**	12×6 = 72

The above tables show us that 12 is the lowest common denominator (LCD). To proceed with the sum, the next stage is to rewrite each fraction in terms of the common denominator, 12ths. So we rewrite $\frac{1}{4}$ in 12ths and $\frac{3}{6}$ in 12ths.

To do this we divide the common denominator 12 by the denominators of the two fractions (4 and 6 in the above example) and then multiply the numerator of each fraction by the respective answer.

We rewrite $\frac{1}{4}$ in 12ths as follows:

$12 \div 4 = 3$ (common denominator $12 \div$ denominator of $4 = 3$)
$3 \times 1 = 3$ (answer $3 \times$ numerator of $1 = 3$)

So we have $\frac{1}{4} = \frac{3}{12}$. Similarly $\frac{3}{6}$ in 12ths is rewritten:

$12 \div 6 = 2$ (common denominator $12 \div$ denominator of $6 = 2$)
$2 \times 3 = 6$ (answer $2 \times$ numerator of $3 = 6$)

So we have $\frac{3}{6} = \frac{6}{12}$.

The sum of $\frac{1}{4} + \frac{3}{6}$ now becomes: $\frac{3}{12} + \frac{6}{12}$. Since these fractions have the same denominator they can be added together as with the previous example:

$$\frac{3}{12} + \frac{6}{12} = \frac{3+6}{12} = \frac{9}{12}$$

Test 13

Work out the lowest common denominator (LCD) of:
1. $\frac{1}{5}$ and $\frac{4}{15}$
2. $\frac{1}{4}$ and $\frac{2}{3}$
3. $\frac{9}{16}$, $\frac{1}{8}$ and $\frac{3}{4}$

Calculate the following using the LCDs above:
4. $\frac{1}{5} + \frac{4}{15}$
5. $\frac{1}{4} + \frac{2}{3}$
6. $\frac{9}{16} - \frac{1}{8}$

Test 14

Work out the LCD and then *choose the larger fraction.* Try to work out the answers 'in your head' as far as possible.

1. $^2/_3$ $^3/_4$ 4. $^3/_4$ $^5/_6$ $^7/_8$
2. $^2/_3$ $^5/_9$ $^{11}/_{18}$ 5. $^{30}/_{100}$ $^7/_{25}$ $^{16}/_{50}$
3. $^1/_3$ $^2/_5$ $^{11}/_{30}$ 6. $^7/_{100}$ $^3/_{50}$ $^{10}/_{1000}$

How to multiply and divide fractions

Multiplication is straightforward. All you have to do is multiply the two numerators (top numbers) together and multiply the two denominators (bottom numbers) together.

Example:

$$\frac{1}{5} \times \frac{2}{3} = \frac{1 \times 2}{5 \times 3} = \frac{2}{15}$$

So when multiplying fractions together the rule is:

Multiply the two top numbers
Multiply the two bottom numbers

Test 15

Calculate the following and cancel the answer where possible:

1. $^2/_3 \times ^1/_9$ 6. $^2/_3 \times ^3/_4$
2. $^4/_{15} \times ^2/_3$ 7. $^3/_5 \times ^5/_9$
3. $^4/_7 \times ^4/_9$ 8. $^7/_{20} \times ^5/_7$
4. $^2/_3 \times ^1/_9$ 9. $^2/_9 \times ^3/_9$
5. $^3/_5 \times ^1/_{100}$ 10. $^9/_{10} \times ^1/_3$

Division of fractions is similar except the fraction on the right-hand side must be:

- turned upside down (e.g. $^3/_5$ becomes $^5/_3$)
- then multiplied with the fraction on the left-hand side.

Example: $\frac{1}{5} \div \frac{3}{10} = ?$

Step one, $\frac{3}{10}$ becomes $\frac{10}{3}$
Step two, $\frac{1}{5} \times \frac{10}{3} = \frac{10}{15}$

So when dividing fractions the rule is:

Turn the right-hand fraction upside down and then multiply the two fractions together.

Test 16

Calculate the following divisions by turning the right-hand side fraction upside down before multiplying the two fractions together.

1.	$\frac{1}{6} \div \frac{1}{4}$	6.	$\frac{12}{100} \div \frac{3}{10}$
2.	$\frac{1}{3} \div \frac{5}{9}$	7.	$\frac{8}{1000} \div \frac{1}{5}$
3.	$\frac{3}{16} \div \frac{1}{4}$	8.	$\frac{1}{250} \div \frac{1}{5}$
4.	$\frac{3}{10} \div \frac{3}{5}$	9.	$\frac{2}{125} \div \frac{8}{75}$
5.	$\frac{5}{12} \div \frac{1}{2}$	10.	$\frac{3}{7} \div \frac{9}{14}$

Improper fractions

Until now, we have worked with fractions that have denominators greater than the numerator (bottom greater than top).

Examples are $\frac{1}{4}$, $\frac{5}{6}$, $\frac{9}{10}$, $\frac{13}{16}$ – these are known as *vulgar fractions*. However, some fractions are *top heavy*, as in $\frac{17}{6}$, $\frac{9}{4}$ and $\frac{65}{25}$. Here the numerator is greater than the denominator. These fractions are known as *improper fractions*, and are added, subtracted, multiplied and divided in the same way as for vulgar fractions.

Example: $\frac{5}{2} + \frac{7}{3} = \frac{15 + 14}{6} = \frac{29}{6}$

Example: $\frac{9}{5} - \frac{10}{6} = \frac{63 + 50}{35} = \frac{13}{35}$

Example: $\frac{9}{4} \times \frac{8}{5} = \frac{72}{20} = \frac{18}{5}$

Example: $\frac{11}{4} \div \frac{9}{7} = \frac{11}{4} \times \frac{7}{9} = \frac{77}{36}$

Test 17

Work out the following sums containing improper fractions, and cancel your answers where possible.

1. $^7/_6 + {}^{11}/_{12}$ 5. $^{12}/_5 + {}^5/_2$
2. $^{14}/_3 - {}^9/_2$ 6. $^5/_3 \times {}^8/_5$
3. $^5/_4 \times {}^3/_2$ 7. $^6/_{25} \div {}^8/_{15}$
4. $^6/_5 \div {}^{12}/_5$ 8. $^{75}/_{20} \times {}^{40}/_3$

Mixed fractions

A mixed fraction consists of a whole number with a vulgar fraction. Examples of mixed fractions are:

$1^1/_2, 2^5/_6, 5^1/_3, 3^3/_4$

To be able to work out sums containing mixed fractions we have to turn the mixed fraction into an improper fraction. To do this, we first separate the whole number from the vulgar fraction, for example:

$1^1/_2$ is one whole and one half: $1 + {}^1/_2$

The next step is to write the whole number in terms of the fraction. In the above example, 1 is 2 halves, so:

$1 = {}^2/_2$

We can now add the whole, expressed as a fraction, to the vulgar fraction:

$1^1/_2 = {}^2/_2 + {}^1/_2 = {}^3/_2$

So $1^1/_2$ as an improper fraction is $^3/_2$.

Similarly, $2^3/_4 = {}^8/_4 + {}^3/_4 = {}^{11}/_4$.

This example can also be shown in diagram form:

$$2\tfrac{3}{4} = \tfrac{11}{4}$$

A more mathematical way of converting a mixed fraction to an improper fraction is as follows:

Step 1: multiply the whole number by the denominator of the vulgar fraction.

Step 2: put the answer in step 1 over the denominator of the vulgar fraction.

Step 3: combine the vulgar fraction with the answer in step 2.

Example: write the mixed fraction $2\tfrac{1}{4}$ as an improper fraction.

Step 1: $2 \times 4 = 8$

Step 2: $\tfrac{8}{4}$ (2 wholes = 8 quarters)

Step 3: $\tfrac{8}{4} + \tfrac{1}{4} = \tfrac{9}{4}$

So $2\tfrac{1}{4}$ as an improper fraction is $\tfrac{9}{4}$.

Test 18

Convert the following mixed fractions to improper fractions and cancel where possible.

1. $1\tfrac{3}{4}$ 4. $3\tfrac{3}{8}$ 7. $1\tfrac{20}{100}$

2. $5\tfrac{1}{2}$ 5. $6\tfrac{7}{10}$ 8. $2\tfrac{10}{25}$

3. $2\tfrac{5}{6}$ 6. $1\tfrac{19}{100}$ 9. $1\tfrac{400}{1000}$

It is also possible to convert an improper fraction into a mixed fraction – the reverse of the above. For example, $\tfrac{27}{8}, \tfrac{9}{2}, \tfrac{7}{3}$ and $\tfrac{11}{10}$ can be converted to mixed fractions. This is done as follows:

Step 1: divide the numerator by the denominator.

Step 2: put the remainder (from the answer in step 1) over the denominator of the improper fraction.

Step 3: combine the whole number (from the answer in step 1) with the answer in step 2.

Example: express the improper fraction $^{21}/_4$ as a mixed fraction.

$$\begin{array}{r} 5 \text{ remainder } \mathbf{1} \\ \text{step (1)} \quad 4\overline{\smash{)}21} \end{array}$$

step (2) $\quad \dfrac{1}{4}$

step (3) combine 5 with $\dfrac{1}{4}$ to give $5\dfrac{1}{4}$

so $\dfrac{21}{4} = 5\dfrac{1}{4}$

Test 19

Convert the following improper fractions to mixed fractions.

1. $^9/_2$ 3. $^{16}/_3$ 5. $^{42}/_8$

2. $^{23}/_4$ 4. $^{50}/_3$ 6. $^{125}/_{10}$

Multiplication and division of fractions by whole numbers

Here it is helpful to rewrite the whole number as *an improper fraction* with a *denominator of 1*, before carrying out the calculation. For example: 2, 3, 4, 5, etc. can be rewritten as

$$\frac{2}{1}, \frac{3}{1}, \frac{4}{1}, \frac{5}{1}$$

Example: $\dfrac{5}{6} \times 2 = \dfrac{5}{6} \times \dfrac{2}{1} = \dfrac{10}{6} = 1\dfrac{4}{6} = 1\dfrac{2}{3}$

□ $\dfrac{5}{6} \times 3 = \dfrac{5}{6} \times \dfrac{3}{1} = \dfrac{15}{6} = 2\dfrac{3}{6} = 2\dfrac{1}{2}$

□ $\dfrac{5}{6} \times 4 = \dfrac{5}{6} \times \dfrac{4}{1} = \dfrac{20}{6} = 3\dfrac{2}{6} = 3\dfrac{1}{3}$

□ $\dfrac{5}{6} \times 5 = \dfrac{5}{6} \times \dfrac{5}{1} = \dfrac{25}{6} = 4\dfrac{1}{6}$

Test 20

Multiply or divide the following fractions by the whole numbers shown and express your answers as mixed fractions.

1. $\frac{1}{2} \times 5$ 5. $^{50}/_{80} \times 12$
2. $\frac{3}{4} \times 6$ 6. $\frac{3}{4} \div 5$
3. $^{7}/_{8} \times 4$ 7. $^{4}/_{9} \div 16$
4. $^{9}/_{5} \times 6$ 8 $^{5}/_{6} \div 20$

How to cross-cancel fractions

Often you can avoid large numbers in nursing calculations by cancelling fractions *diagonally* rather than just top and bottom. Cross-cancelling in this way helps to simplify the arithmetic.

Example: $^{7}/_{8} \times ^{9}/_{14}$ without cross-cancelling becomes $^{63}/_{112}$. In cross-cancelling, the 7 can be cancelled diagonally with the 14 (7 goes into 7 once and 7 goes into 14 twice). The calculation then becomes: $^{1}/_{8} \times ^{9}/_{2}$ giving $^{9}/_{16}$ as the answer.

Example: $^{8}/_{15} \times ^{5}/_{16}$ without cross-cancelling becomes $^{40}/_{240}$. In cross-cancelling, the 8 can be cancelled diagonally with the 16, and the 5 can be cancelled diagonally with the 15. The calculation becomes $^{1}/_{3} \times ^{1}/_{2}$ giving $^{1}/_{6}$ as the answer.

It is difficult to cross-cancel 'in your head' so you would normally write the calculation as follows:

$$\overset{1}{\underset{3}{\cancel{\frac{8}{15}}}} \times \overset{1}{\underset{2}{\cancel{\frac{5}{16}}}} = \frac{1}{3} \times \frac{1}{2} = \frac{1}{6}$$

Test 21

Work out the following by cross-cancelling as a first step. Express your answers as mixed fractions or whole numbers.

1. $^7/_3 \times {}^3/_5$ 3. $^{240}/_{50} \times {}^5/_3$ 5. $^{32}/_{40} \times 80$
2. $^{51}/_{16} \times {}^4/_3$ 4. $^3/_{10} \times 100$ 6. $^{36}/_{500} \times 1000$

(In the following divisions, cross-cancel after turning the right-hand side number upside down).

7. $^5/_{12} \div {}^{16}/_{24}$ 10. $^{40}/_{150} \div {}^{64}/_{120}$ 13. $^3/_4 \div {}^{375}/_{100}$
8. $^{17}/_{100} \div {}^{34}/_{50}$ 11. $^{100}/_{480} \div {}^{110}/_{132}$ 14. $^{48}/_{60} \div {}^{80}/_{360}$
9. $^{27}/_{100} \div {}^3/_5$ 12. $^{14}/_{216} \div {}^{28}/_{36}$ 15. $^{15}/_{100} \div 60$

Test 22

Work out the following by first converting the mixed fractions to improper fractions. The answers are all whole numbers.

1. $4^1/_2 \times {}^2/_3$ 4. $20 \div 2^1/_2$ 7. $5^1/_4 \div 1^3/_4$
2. $2^4/_5 \times 5$ 5. $1^1/_3 \div {}^1/_6$ 8. $^{45}/_{100} \times {}^{22}/_9$
3. $4^4/_9 \times 1^4/_5$ 6. $2^2/_3 \div {}^8/_{15}$ 9. $1^{200}/_{1000} \times 4^1/_6$

Introduction to decimals

Decimal numbers are numbers that contain a decimal point. *Decimal fractions* are decimal numbers smaller than one (nought point something); they are fractions of a whole number. The decimal point (.) separates the whole number from the fraction.

Decimal in words	Decimal in figures			
	Units	Tenths	Hun.ths	Thou.ths
three point five eight	3.	5	8	
one point two five six	1.	2	5	6
nought point seven three	0.	7	3	

Necessary and unnecessary zeros

It is important to understand which zeros are needed and which are not when writing both whole numbers and decimals. Whole numbers such as 2, 10 and 250 should not be written as 2.0, 10.0 and 250.0 – the decimal point and 0 after it are unnecessary and could lead to errors if misread as 20, 100 and 2500. For a similar reason, a 0 should always be placed in front of the decimal point when there is no other number (example: write 0.73 not .73).
The following are examples of unnecessary zeros:

0.30	0.300	0.3000	which should all be written as 0.3
0.850	0.8500	0.850 00	which should be written as 0.85

The following are examples of necessary zeros:

0.3	0.03	0.003	which all have different values
0.802	0.8002	0.800 02	which all have different values

Test 23

Write out the following numbers in figures
1. twenty two point five
2. nought point two seven five
3. nought point nought two
4. two hundred point zero seven five

Place the numbers (in columns a, b, c and d) in order of size, starting with the *smallest first*. Write a, b, c, d. Take your time and double check.

	(a)	(b)	(c)	(d)
5.	2.5	0.25	0.3	0.025
6.	0.05	0.1	0.08	0.75
7.	3.025	3.25	3.05	3.04
8.	6.20	6.02	6.026	6.22
9.	10.01	10.101	10.011	10.11

Multiplication by powers of 10 x 10, x 100, x 1000)

To multiply a decimal number by 10, 100, 1000, etc., you just move the decimal point to the right by however many powers of 10 you have – or put another way, by how many 0s you have (a calculator is not required). To multiply:

x 10 you move the decimal point one place to the right.
x 100 you move the decimal point two places to the right.
x 1000 you move the decimal point three places to the right.

For example: what is 5.178 × 100?

Answer: 5.178 × 100 = 517.8
Similarly: 0.0235 × 10 = 0.235

Division by powers of 10 (÷ 10, ÷ 100, ÷ 1000)

Just as in the multiplication of decimals, you can divide decimals by powers of 10 (10, 100, 1000 etc) by moving the decimal point. This is simply the reverse of the multiplication case so when dividing you move the decimal point to the left.

Example:

25.34 ÷ 10 = 2.534
     ÷ 100 = 0.2534
     ÷ 1000 = 0.02534

Other examples are:

256.98 ÷ 100 = 2.5698
       ÷ 1000 = 0.25698

Similarly: 0.0037 ÷ 100 = 0.000 037.

Test 24

Work out the following multiplications and divisions. Hint: the number of 0s following the 1 is the number of places to move the decimal point – either to the right (to multiply) or to the left (to divide).

1. $1.5897 \times 1000 =$
2. $7\ 692\ 105 \div 10000 =$
3. $31.729 \times 100 =$
4. $0.175 \div 10 =$
5. $17.1703 \times 1000 =$
6. $0.025 \times 1000 =$
7. $0.0058 \times 1000 =$
8. $0.0001 \times 1\ 000\ 000 =$

Addition, subtraction, multiplication and division of decimals

The addition and subtraction of decimal numbers is the same as for ordinary numbers. The only thing to remember is to keep the decimal points aligned. Adding unnecessary 0s can help.

Example: $0.36 + 0.28 + 0.052 + 0.1$

```
0.360
0.280
0.052
0.100 +
0.792
```

The multiplication of decimals is similar to the multiplication of whole numbers, with an extra step to work out the position of the decimal point. The 'golden rule' to find the position is:

Number of decimal places (dp) in the question = Number of dp in answer

Example:

4.21	two decimal places	
3	× no decimal places	
12.63	two decimal places in the answer	

Example: 0.002×0.03

0.002	three decimal places
0.03 ×	two decimal places
0.000 06	five decimal places in the answer

Note that all unnecessary 0s should be removed before you multiply the numbers together.

Test 25

Multiply the following decimal numbers. Treat these as whole numbers first and then add the decimal point as a second step.
1. 3.2×2.8
2. 3.08×6.5
3. 0.095×3.74
4. 0.002×2.72 (handy hint: place the 0.002 below the 2.72)
5. 10.01×0.15
6. 500×0.32 (handy hint: multiply 0.32 by 100 and then by 5)
7. 75×0.04
8. 33.4×3
9. 800×2.54 (handy hint: multiply 2.54 by 100 and then by 8)
10. 4000×3.50

The division of decimal numbers is carried out in the same way as with whole numbers, leaving the decimal point in the same position.

Example: $24.369 \div 3$

8.123	keep the decimal point in
3⟌24.369	the same position when
	dividing a decimal number

If the number that you are dividing by contains a decimal point, for example 0.35 or 3.5, then it must be converted to a whole number before the division can take place. To do this you must multiply both numbers by a power of 10 – by 10, 100, 1000, etc. – to remove the decimal point from the number that you are dividing by.

Example: $4.5 \div 0.3$ becomes $45 \div 3$ by multiplying both of numbers by 10 to remove the decimal point from the 0.3.

Similarly: $9.375 \div 0.02$ becomes $937.5 \div 2$ by multiplying both of the numbers by 100 to remove the decimal point from the 0.02.

These divisions can now be carried out as if they were whole numbers.

Test 26

Work out the following divisions involving decimal numbers. If the number you are *dividing* by contains a decimal point this must be removed first (questions 4 to 11).

1.	$6.8 \div 4$	7.	$3.6 \div 0.6$
2.	$62.25 \div 5$	8.	$9 \div 0.15$
3.	$64.25 \div 8$	9.	$1.44 \div 1.2$
4.	$6.8 \div 0.04$	10.	$125 \div 0.002$
5.	$9.99 \div 0.3$	11.	$1000 \div 0.05$
6.	$5.55 \div 0.50$	12.	$0.08 \div 5$

How to round decimal numbers

Sometimes the numbers you obtain from a calculation are longer than is required for a sensible answer. Example: $3.75 \times 4.01 = 15.0375$. If this level of *accuracy* is not required, you can shorten the number by *rounding it off*. To do this you decrease the number of numbers to the right of the decimal point – that is, you decrease the number of decimal places (dp).

For example, a number such as 15.0375 that has four dp (four numbers to the right of the decimal point) can be rounded off so that it has three, two or one dp.

Method

If the number to the right of the decimal place you are shortening to is 5 or more, then you increase the number in the decimal place by 1; if is less than 5 it remains the same.

Example: round off 15.0375 to three dp – that is, to three numbers to the right of the decimal point.
   Answer: The number to the right of the third dp is 5 (15.0375) so we increase the number in the third dp by 1.

15.0375 becomes 15.038.
15.0375 = 15.038 correct to three dp.

Other examples are:

Round off 15.0375 to two dp
Answer: 15.0375 to two dp = 15.04
Round off 15.0375 to one dp
Answer: 15.0375 to one dp = 15.0

Round off 1.976 to 1 decimal place

more than 5 so the
9 becomes a 10 (1 unit)
Answer 1.976 to 1 decimal place = 2.0

Test 27

From the five alternatives choose *one*.
1. 6.08323 to 2 decimal places is:

| 6.083 | 6.08 | 6.0 | 6.0832 | 6.09 |

2. 0.385426 to 5 decimal places is:

| 0.38543 | 0.39 | 0.3854 | 0.385 | 0.4 |

3. 0.754 to 1 decimal place is is:

    0.75   0.7   0.754   0.8   1.0

4. 7.956 to 2 decimal places is:

    7.95   8.0   7.96   7.0   7.956

Test 28

Work out the following and then give your answer to the number of dp shown.

1. $25 \div 6 =$ (to two dp)
2. $100 \div 7 =$ (to four dp)
3. $3.45 \times 3 =$ (to one dp)
4. $14.5 \times 3 =$ (to the nearest whole number = to 0 dp)

Work out the following and then give your answer to the nearest whole number.

5. $325 \div 4 =$ 8. $100 \div 6$
6. $1279 \div 8 =$ 9. $73 \div 22$
7. $655 \div 10 =$ 10. $400 \div 3$

Conversion of decimals to fractions

In order to convert a decimal to a fraction you divide the numbers to the right of the decimal point by:

10 if one number is present
100 if two numbers are present
1000 if three numbers are present, etc.

Then cancel the fraction to its lowest terms.

For example: $0.5 = {}^{5}/_{10} = {}^{1}/_{2}$
                  $0.25 = {}^{25}/_{100} = {}^{1}/_{4}$
                  $0.125 = {}^{125}/_{1000} = {}^{1}/_{8}$

Test 29

Convert the following decimal numbers to fractions using the method outlined above.

1.	0.6	4.	0.9	7.	0.95
2.	0.75	5.	0.001	8.	1.75
3.	0.625	6.	0.08	9.	2.375

Conversion of fractions to decimals

In nursing and scientific work it is usually more convenient to express a fraction as a decimal. The method is straightforward. All you have to do is divide the denominator (bottom number) into the numerator (top number).

Example: Express $\frac{1}{2}$ as a decimal number.

First step: rewrite $\frac{1}{2}$ as $2\overline{)1}$

Second step: rewrite the 1 as 1.0000 by adding a string of zeros.

$$2\overline{)1.0000}$$

This division is carried out in the same way as with ordinary numbers, leaving the decimal point in the same position.

2 into 1 won't go so you put a 0 down and carry the 1 into the next column to make 10. 2 into 10 goes 5 times.

$$\begin{array}{r} 0.5 \\ 2\overline{)1.^{1}0000} \end{array}$$

So $\frac{1}{2}$ expressed as a decimal number is 0.5.

Example: $\frac{5}{8}$ as a decimal $= 8\overline{)5.0000}$

$$\begin{array}{r} 0.6\ 2\ 5 \\ = 8\overline{)5.^{5}0^{2}0^{4}00} \end{array}$$

$$= 0.625.$$

Example: $\frac{7}{400}$ as a decimal $= 400\overline{)7.0000}$

$$\begin{array}{r} 0.0\ 1\ \ 7\ \ 5 \\ = 400\overline{)7.^{7}00^{300}0^{200}0} \end{array}$$

$$= 0.0175$$

Test 30

Express the following fractions as decimal numbers:

1. $^3/_{10}$ 4. $^5/_4$ 7. $^{17}/_{20}$
2. $^1/_4$ 5. $^3/_{25}$ 8. $^{21}/_{200}$
3. $^2/_5$ 6. $^7/_8$ 9. $^{27}/_{150}$

How to work out percentages

A percentage (the percentage sign is %) means 'out of 100': in other words something is split into 100 equal parts and each one part is 1 per cent. A percentage is basically a special case of a fraction. *All* percentage fractions have the same bottom number, which is 100. All that changes is the top number.

For example: 3% = (3 ÷ 100) 99% = (99 ÷ 100)

A percentage fraction can be cancelled to its lowest terms:

40% = (40 ÷ 100) which cancels to $^4/_{10}$ and finally to $^2/_5$
12% = (12 ÷ 100) which cancels to $^6/_{50}$ and finally to $^3/_{25}$

Percentages can also be written in decimal form. To do this we divide the percentage by 100, expressing the answer as a decimal. The easiest way to divide by 100 is to move the decimal point two places to the left.

Example: 40% as a decimal.   40.0 ÷ 100 = 0.4

Example: 99% as a decimal.   99.0 ÷ 100 = 0.99

Example: 3% as a decimal.   03.0 ÷ 100 = 0.03

Test 31

Convert the following percentages to both fractions and decimals.

1. 20%	4. 75%	7. 35%
2. 25%	5. 90%	8. 22%
3. 10%	6. 45%	9. 2%

How do you work out the percentage of something? To do this you must multiply the 'something' by the percentage fraction.

Example: find 25% of 60.

First step: $25\% = {}^{25}/_{100} = {}^{1}/_{4}$
Second step: $^{1}/_{4} \times 60 = {}^{60}/_{4} = 15$

Another method is to convert the percentage to a decimal fraction as a first step.

Example: find 25% of 60

First step: $25\% = 25 \div 100 = 0.25$
Second step: $0.25 \times 60 = 15$

In the above example, the fraction method of working out the answer was easier than the decimal method, but in some cases the reverse is true.

Test 32

Work out the following percentages using either the fractions method (questions 1 and 2) or the decimal method (questions 3 and 4).

1. 50% of 180
2. 30% of 200
3. 62.5% of 200
4. 212% of 1000
5. If 90% of nursing school applicants fail to become nurses what percentage are successful?
6. If there are 90 000 applicants how many will become nurses?

How to express numbers as percentages

We have seen that percentage means out of 100, so:

$100\% = {}^{100}/_{100} = 1$

This means that we can write any number as a percentage, without affecting its value, by multiplying it by 100% ($\times$ 1).

Whole numbers can be converted to percentages as follows:

Example: $2 \times 100\% = 200\%$ (2 wholes is 200%)
Similarly: $10 \times 100\% = 1000\%$ (10 wholes is 1000%)

Fractions can be converted to percentages in the same way:

Example: $\frac{1}{4} \times 100\% = 25\%$ similarly ${}^{3}/_{10} \times 100\% = 30\%$

Decimal fractions can be converted to percentages in the same way, by multiplying by 100%, for example:

$0.15 \times 100\% = 15\%$ $0.01 \times 100\% = 1\%$
$0.995 \times 100\% = 99.5\%$ $1.1 \times 100\% = 110\%$

Test 33

Convert each decimal or fraction to a percentage by multiplying it by 100%.

1. 0.5
2. 0.75
3. 1.0
4. $\frac{1}{5}$
5. $\frac{1}{8}$

6. 0.015
7. 1.05
8. 0.005
9. $\frac{9}{25}$
10. $\frac{17}{20}$

Chapter 2 questions

Target = 18 correct answers out of 20 questions.

1. $\frac{1}{5} + \frac{2}{5} =$
2. $\frac{5}{9} - \frac{3}{9} =$
3. $\frac{3}{4} \times \frac{1}{2} =$
4. $\frac{3}{7} \div \frac{3}{2} =$
5. $\frac{5}{32} - \frac{1}{8} =$
6. Cancel $\frac{35}{100}$
7. Convert $\frac{27}{7}$ to a mixed fraction.
8. Convert $4\frac{1}{2}$ to an improper fraction.
9. $\frac{7}{8} \times 7 =$
10. $\frac{3}{10} \div 6 =$
11. Place the following numbers in order of increasing size: 3/4, 0.625, 1.2, 0.905, 0.95
12. 1.5 + 0.75 − 0.05 =
13. Multiply 0.005 by 1000.
14. Multiply 0.8 by 0.9.
15. Divide 62.5 by 1000.
16. Divide 25 by 0.005.
17. Write 8.375 to two dp.
18. Convert $\frac{1}{6}$ to a decimal number; give your answer to 3 dp.
19. Convert 0.0625 to a fraction.
20. What is 5% of 250?

3 Measurement

The metric system of measurement (SI units)

You will need to familiarise yourself with the metric system of measurements as appropriate to nursing, the most important of which are weight and volume. SI units (international system) are in most cases the same as metric units, all being based on units of 10.

Weight

The basic unit of weight is the gram (g). All metric weights are based on this. There are four weights you are likely to encounter:

Name	Symbol
kilogram	kg
gram	g
milligram	mg
microgram	mcg

One kilogram is equivalent to 1000 grams.

1 kg = 1000 g and 1g = $\frac{1}{1000}$ th of a kg.

One gram is equivalent to 1000 mg.

1 g = 1000 mg and 1 mg = $\frac{1}{1000}$ th of a g.

One milligram is equivalent to 1000 mcg.

1 mg = 1000 mcg and 1 mcg = $\frac{1}{1000}$ th of a mg.

We have abbreviated microgram to mcg in preference to µg which can be confused with mg with untidy handwriting when the 'µ' looks like an 'm'. *Confusion can be avoided by writing out the word microgram in full instead of using abbreviations.*

In some calculations it is necessary to convert from one unit of weight to another, for example, grams to milligrams, kilograms to grams.

For example: convert 2 g to milligrams. Since 1 g = 1000 mg, to convert grams to milligrams you multiply by 1000. So 2 g in milligrams is 2 × 1000 = 2000 mg.

Similarly 5.5 kg converted to g is 5.5 × 1000 = 5500 g.

Another example: convert 2200 mg to grams. This time we divide by 1000 because 1 mg = $\frac{1}{1000}$th of a gram. So 2200 mg in grams is 2200 ÷ 1000 = 2.2 g.

To convert grams to micrograms you use two steps:

Step 1, convert grams to milligrams.

Step 2, convert milligrams to micrograms.

For example: convert 1.5 g to micrograms.

Step 1: 1.5 g = 1.5 × 1000 mg = 1500 mg.
Step 2: 1500 mg = 1500 × 1000 mcg = 1 500 000 mcg.
So 1.5 g = 1 500 000 micrograms.

From this we can see that one microgram is one thousandth of a milligram and therefore one millionth of a gram, or put another way, there are one million micrograms in one gram.

Choosing the best units for your answer

It is important to choose the most appropriate units for your answer when working with metric quantities. An answer worked out as 1 500 000 micrograms should be written as 1.5 g to avoid a long string of zeros. Similarly an answer of 1500 mg would also be expressed as 1.5 g. However, 0.15 g should be written as 150 mg to avoid the use of a decimal point; similarly 0.15 mg should be expressed as 150 micrograms for the same reason. The following guidelines should be adopted when choosing units.

Guidelines for choosing units of weight

Answers of less than 1 kg (1000 g) are written in grams, for example: 1.5 g, 2.25 g, 20 g, 275 g, 750.5 g, 950g.

Answers of less than 1 g (1000 mg) are written in milligrams, for example: 1.25 mg, 2.5 mg, 50 mg, 75.1 mg, 450.5 mg.

Answers of less than 1 mg (1000 microgram) are written in micrograms, for example: 2 micrograms, 50 micrograms, 125 micrograms, 750 micrograms.

Answers such as 0.5 mg are non-standard and should be written as 500 micrograms to avoid using a decimal point. However 0.5 can be retained when expressing a range such as 0.5–1 g. The decimal point should always have a leading zero if no whole number is present, so write 0.5 not .5, where the decimal point can easily be missed.

Test 34

Convert the following weights to the metric units specified by moving the decimal point.
1. 0.025 mg to micrograms
2. 0.001 kg to grams
3. 0.33 mg to micrograms
4. 1275 mg to grams
5. 420 micrograms to mg

Test 35

Express the following metric quantities in the best units (kg, g, mg or micrograms).

1.	1000 mg =	7.	325 micrograms =
2.	2500 mg =	8.	10 000 micrograms =
3.	1250 mg =	9.	1200 g =
4.	4500 micrograms =	10.	0.05 g =
5.	0.5 g =	11.	0.5 mg
6.	0.25 g =	12.	0.000012 g

Volume

Quantities of liquids are measured in litres (L). You are probably familiar with litres through putting fuel in your car. In nursing you will also meet the millilitre (mL or ml: both can be used but mL is more common in nursing).
A litre is 1000 millilitres:

1 L = 1000 mL and 1 mL = $\frac{1}{1000}$ th of 1 L

Test 36

Convert the following volumes to the metric units specified by moving the decimal point.

1. 0.5 L to mL
2. 0.05 L to mL
3. 1.25 L to mL
4. 0.125 L to mL
5. 2000 mL to L
6. 4050 mL to L
7. 5 mL to L
8. 250 mL to L
9. 10.5 mL to L
10. 0.01 L to mL

Test 37

Complete the following review of metric quantities. All of your answers should be *symbols*.

1. kilogram is ...
2. litre is ...
3. milligram is ...
4. microgram is ... or ...
5. 1 gram × 1000 = 1 ...
6. 1 milligram × 1000 = 1 ...
7. 1 milligram ÷ 1000 = 1 ...
8. 1 microgram × 1 000 000 = 1...
9. 1 millilitre × 1000 = 1 ...

Test 38

Add or subtract the following metric quantities and give your answer in the units shown in the brackets. Hint: the first step is to convert everything to the units stated.

1. 1.6 g + 500 mg (in g)
2. 1.6 g + 50 mg (in g)
3. 2.75 g + 250 mg (in g)
4. 1.2 g – 500 mg (in g)
5. 0.6 mg + 300 micrograms (in mg)
6. 0.01 mg + 425 micrograms (in micrograms)
7. 0.5 g + 100 mg + 500 micrograms (in g)
8. 750 mcg – 0.075 mg (in micrograms)

Test 39

Multiply or divide the following metric quantities and give your answer in the units specified. Hint: carry out the multiplication first and then convert to the units shown in the brackets afterwards. The 'speed tip' will help you with the multiplication.

1. 25 mg × 40 (in g) speed tip: 25 × 40 = 25 × 4 × 10
2. 75 mg × 20 (in g) speed tip: 75 × 20 = 75 × 2 × 10
3. 50 mcg × 250 (in mg) speed tip: 50 × 250 = 100 × 125
4. 125 mcg × 16 (in mg) speed tip: 125 × 16 = 250 × 8 = 500 × 4
5. 250 g × 1.2 (in kg) speed tip: 250 × 1.2 = 25 × 12 = 100 × 3

Hint: convert to the units shown in the brackets first and then carry out the division.

6. 1 g ÷ 200 (in mg)
7. 10 mg ÷ 50 (in micrograms)
8. 1.5 mg ÷ 200 (in micrograms)
9. 0.004 mg ÷ 8 (in micrograms)
10. 1 kg ÷ 400 (in g)

Time

You should be aware that:

60 seconds (sec) = 1 minute (min)
60 minutes = 1 hour (hr, h)
24 hours = 1 day (d)
7 days = 1 week (wk)
52 weeks = 1 year (yr)
am = before noon (midday); pm = afternoon

Candidates should be familiar with both the 12-hour clock (which has two 12-hour periods – am and pm) and the 24-hour clock which starts and finishes at midnight (00:00/24:00 hrs). Noon (midday) = 12:00 hrs (twelve hundred hours). Times can be converted from the 12-hour clock to the 24-hour clock by rewriting the time as a four-digit number and adding 12 hours to all pm times.

Examples: 8.30 am = 08:30 hrs (zero eight thirty hours)
1 pm = 1 + 12 = 13:00 hrs (thirteen hundred hours)
10.45 pm = 10.45 + 12 = 22:45 hrs (twenty two forty five hours)

Likewise, times on the 24-hour clock can be converted to 12-hour clock times by subtracting 12 hours from all afternoon times (those greater than 12:00 hrs).

Example: 20:50 hrs = 20:50 − 12:00 = 8.50 pm
You should be able to convert any fraction of an hour into minutes and any fraction of a minute into seconds.

Examples: $\frac{1}{2}$ hour = 30 minutes
$\frac{1}{4}$ hour = 15 minutes
$\frac{1}{3}$ minute = 20 seconds

Additional examples are:

$\frac{1}{10}$ th hour = $\frac{1}{10} \times \frac{60}{1}$ minutes = 6 minutes
$\frac{3}{5}$ th minute = $\frac{3}{5} \times \frac{1}{60}$ seconds = 3 x12 = 36 seconds
$2\frac{5}{6}$ th hours = 2 + ($\frac{5}{6} \times \frac{1}{60}$) minutes = 2 hrs 50 minutes
0.75 hours = 0.75 × 60 minutes = 45 minutes
0.2 hours = 0.2 × 60 minutes = 12 minutes
2.4 hours = 2 + (0.4 × 60) minutes = 2 hrs 24 minutes

Test 40

Work out following clock times and complete the calculations involving measurements of time.
1. Write 6.25 am as a 24-hour clock time
2. Write 5.05 pm as a 24-hour clock time
3. Write 21:50 hrs as a 12-hour clock time
4. Write 10:10 hrs as a 12-hour clock time
5. What time is it when 1.5 hours is added to 6 pm?
6. What time is it when 3.25 hours is added to 22:30 hours?
7. Write 93 minutes in hours and minutes
8. Convert 0.3 hours to minutes
9. Convert 2.2 minutes to seconds
10. Express 40 seconds as a fraction of 1 minute
11. How many seconds are there in 0.9 minutes?
12. How many seconds are there in 0.33 minutes? (give your answer to the nearest second)

Reading instrument scales

A scale is a set of marks on a line used for measuring. Examples are found on rulers, measuring jugs, blood pressure gauges and patients' observation charts. Scales usually have regular spaces (intervals) between the 'tick marks' (*graduation* lines), for example, millimetres on rulers. Most scales begin at zero with the graduation lines spread evenly along the length. Other scales are circular with the graduation spread evenly around a dial, as seen on a blood pressure gauge.

The key to reading any scale is in knowing how many intervals there are between the numbers. The metric system is based on units of 10, and metric scales normally have 10 intervals. A 15 cm ruler, for example, has each centimetre divided into 10 millimetres. Here are some examples of graduated scales.

Measuring jug: 750 mL full (halfway between 700 and 800 mL):

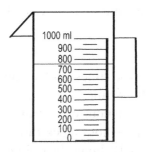

Measuring jug: 50 mL full (halfway between 0 and 100 mL):

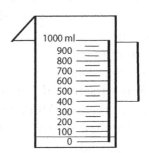

Graduated syringes (not drawn to scale):

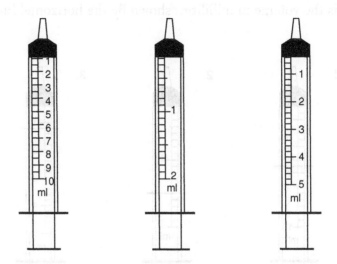

On the 10 mL syringe on the left there are two graduations for every 1 mL, so each graduation mark represents 0.5 mL (each mL is divided into two equal parts).

On the 2 mL syringe in the middle there are 10 graduations for every 1 mL, so each graduation mark represent 0.1 mL (each mL is divided into 10 equal parts).

On the 5 mL syringe on the right there are five graduations for every 1 mL, so each graduation mark represent 0.2 mL (each mL is divided into five equal parts).

Use the above information to work out the volume of solution in each of the 12 syringes shown on the following pages. Some of the syringes are of 1 mL capacity, and as a first step you will need to work out the volume represented by one graduation mark using the method outlined above.

Test 41

What is the volume in millilitres shown by the horizontal line?

1. 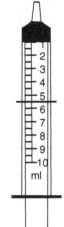   **2.** 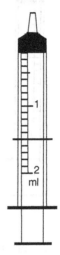   **3.**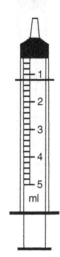

4. 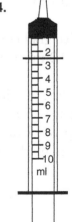   **5.** 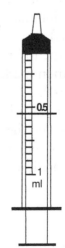   **6.**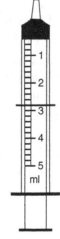

Test 42

What is the volume in millilitres shown by the horizontal line?

1.

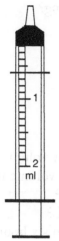

2.

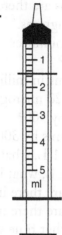

3.

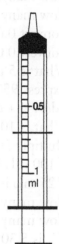

4.

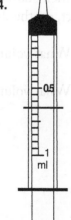

5.

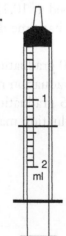

6.

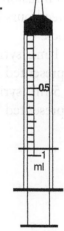

Chapter 3 questions

1. How many grams are there in 2000 milligrams?
2. How many milligrams are there in 0.4 g?
3. How many micrograms are there in 0.25 mg?
4. How many micrograms are there in 0.01 mg?
5. Convert 0.08 g to milligrams.
6. Convert 0.0075 L to millilitres.
7. What is 5 g + 500 mg?
8. Express 950 micrograms in milligrams.
9. Add 7 g + 654 mg + 320 micrograms?
10. What is 10 g divided by 500?
11. Multiply 500 micrograms by 300.
12. If 100 mL is added to 1 L, what is the new volume in litres?
13. If 25 mL is added to 1 L, what is the new volume in litres?
14. How many millilitres are there in 0.062 L?
15. How many millilitres are there in 0.5775 L?
16. If it is 5.30 pm now, what time will it be in six hours on the 24-hour clock?
17. If it is 8.30 pm now, what time will it be in 12 hours on the 24-hour clock?
18. An infusion was stopped at 10.15 am and then started again three hours later. At what time did it restart, on the 24-hour clock?
19. A 1 mL syringe has 20 graduation marks. What volume is represented by each graduation mark?
20. A 5 mL syringe has 25 graduation marks. What volume is represented by 20 graduation marks?

4 Drug dosage calculations

Oral medications

The easiest drug calculations to perform are those that involve oral medications. These medications are usually dispensed as tablets or capsules, or sometimes as liquids if the patient has difficulty swallowing or is a child.

Calculations for tablets involve wholes. For example, 1 gram of paracetamol requires two 500 milligram tablets; only scored tablets may be split in half. Most liquid medications (syrups, elixirs, solutions, suspensions, mixtures, linctuses and emulsions) are measured out in millilitres, using a graduated measuring cup, spoon or syringe.

There is a general equation that applies to all oral medications; whether in tablet or liquid form:

$$\text{Amount required} = \frac{\text{Strength required}}{\text{Stock strength}} \times \text{volume of stock strength}$$

For calculating the number of tablets, the formula can be rewritten as:

Number of tablets = $\dfrac{\text{Dose prescribed}}{\text{Dose per tablet}}$

Example: A dose of 15 mg of a drug is prescribed. This drug is supplied in 5 mg tablets. How many tablets are given?

$$= \frac{15 \text{ mg}}{5 \text{ mg}} = 3 \text{ tablets}$$

Key point: You must make sure that the units are the same for both the prescribed dosage and dosage per tablet.

Example: 1.2 grams of a drug is prescribed. Each tablet contains 600 mg of the drug. How many tablets are to be dispensed?

Note that the units are not the same (grams and milligrams) so we need to convert one unit into the other unit as a first step. In most cases it is easiest to convert the bigger unit into the smaller unit, so convert grams into milligrams. We do this by multiplying by 1000.

First step: 1.2 g = 1.2 × 1000 = 1200 mg (see the metric system).

Second step:

2nd step: **Number of tablets** = $\dfrac{\text{Dose prescribed}}{\text{Dose per tablet}}$

$$= \frac{1200 \text{ mg}}{600 \text{ mg}} = 2 \text{ tablets}$$

For calculating the amount of liquid to be administered, the formula can be written as:

Amount required = $\dfrac{\text{Dose prescribed}}{\text{Stock strength}}$ x volume of stock strength

Example: a syrup is prescribed. The syrup has 4 mg of drug per 5 mL liquid. If the patient needs 12 mg, how much syrup should be administered by graduated medicine cup?

The measure in this case is a volume of drug so the equation can be rewritten as:

Amount required $= \dfrac{\text{Dose prescribed}}{\text{Dose per ml}}$ x volume of stock strength

$= \dfrac{12 \text{ mg} \times 5 \text{ ml}}{4 \text{ mg}}$

$= 15 \text{ mL}$

Example: a patient needs 50 mg of a drug. The stock bottle contains 25 mg per 5 mL. How many mL should be measured out?

Amount required $= \dfrac{\text{Dose prescribed}}{\text{Stock strength}}$ x volume of stock strength

$= \dfrac{50 \text{ mg}}{25 \text{ mg}} \times 5 \text{ ml}$

$= 2 \times 5 \text{ ml} = 10 \text{ ml}$

Example: a patient needs 300 mg of a drug. If the stock bottle contains 100 mg in 10 mL, how many mL should be drawn up?

$$\textbf{Number of mL} = \frac{\text{Dose prescribed}}{\text{Dose per measure}} \times \text{Volume of stock strength}$$

$$= \frac{300 \text{ mg}}{100 \text{ mg}} \times 10 \text{ mL} = 3 \times 10 \text{ mL} = 30 \text{ mL}$$

You can check your answer as follows: 30 mL = 3 lots of 10 mL; 3 lots of 100 mg = 300 mg (correct dose).

Test 43

No of Measures = Dose Prescribed ÷ Dose per Measure

1. A drug in tablet form is prescribed. The required dosage is 75 mg. The tablets are in 25 mg each. How many tablets should be dispensed?
2. The patient is written up for 500 micrograms of a drug and each tablet contains 0.25 mg. How many tablets are required?
3. 30 mg of a drug is prescribed. The drug is in liquid form and is to be given orally. It has strength of 10 mg per 5 mL. What volume is dispensed?
4. 60 mg of a drug is prescribed. The drug is in liquid form and is to be given orally. The strength is 30 mg/5 mL. What volume is dispensed?
5. A patient requires 20 mg of a drug in liquid form. If the stock contains 10 mg in 2 mL, what volume of the drug should be drawn up?
6. 1.5 milligrams of a drug are prescribed. Each tablet contains 500 micrograms. How many tablets should be dispensed?
7. A patient requires 500 micrograms of a drug and each tablet contains 0.125 mg. How many tablets are required?
8. A patient requires 200 micrograms of a drug orally. The stock contains 0.1 mg in 5 mL. How much liquid should be administered?

9. The bottle contains 100 milligrams of a drug per 5 mL. What dose will the patient receive if 20 mL is measured out?
10. The stock contains 250 micrograms per 2 mL. What dose will the patient receive if 10 mL is measured out?

Injections

Drugs for injection are usually supplied in ampoules or vials. Glass ampoules have to be broken off at the neck. The ampoule is inverted to an angle of 45 degrees and the solution is withdrawn with a needle and syringe. Glass vials, with rubber stoppers, often contain a drug in powdered form which has to be reconstituted with a diluent, typically sterile Water for Injection BP, before use.

A needle and syringe are used to add the water to the vial and the mixture is shaken to reconstitute the drug. To withdraw the solution, the equivalent volume of air is pushed into the vial. The reconstituted drug is then drawn up into the syringe (*aspirated*). Some powdered drugs displace water, in which case the volume of water to add is always less than the final volume in the vial. For example: to make 10 mL of solution add 9.8 mL of sterilised water. Here the *displacement volume* is 0.2 mL.

Calculating drug dosages for injection is very similar to calculating oral doses. However, the dose prescribed is often less than the dose in stock, so you must be able to cancel fractions to their lowest terms and also be able to convert fractions to decimals.

Example: a vial contains 1 mg of a drug in 10 mL of solution. How many millilitres need to be drawn up for a dose of:

a) 500 micrograms?   b) 50 micrograms?
c) 250 micrograms?   d) 1500 micrograms?

The first step is to convert the 1 mg dose to micrograms:

1 mg = 1 × 1000 micrograms = 1000 micrograms

The second step uses the equation:

$$\text{Number of mL} = \frac{\text{Dose prescribed}}{\text{Dose per measure}} \times 10 \text{ mL}$$

a) Number of mL = $^{500}/_{1000} \times 10$ mL = $^1/_2 \times {^{10}/_1} = {^{10}/_2} = 5$ mL

(Method: cancel the fraction to its lowest terms, multiply it by 10 and convert the improper fraction to a whole number.)

b) Number of mL = $^{50}/_{1000} \times 10$ mL = $^1/_{20} \times {^{10}/_1} = {^{10}/_{20}} = {^1/_2} = 0.5$ mL

(Method: cancel the fraction to its lowest terms, multiply it by 10, cancel the fraction to its lowest terms and convert it to a decimal number.)

c) Number of mL = $^{250}/_{1000} \times 10$ mL = $^1/_4 \times {^{10}/_1} = {^{10}/_4} = {^5/_2} = 2.5$ mL

(Method: same as in b.)

d) Number of mL = $^{1500}/_{1000} \times 10$ mL = $^3/_2 \times {^{10}/_1} = {^{30}/_2} = 15$ mL

(Method: cancel the improper fraction to its lowest terms, multiply it by 10 and cancel the improper fraction to its lowest terms.)

Test 44

1. An oral solution contains 100 mg of drug in every 5 mL. How many mL must be drawn up for a dose of:
    a) 10 mg   b) 15 mg   c) 20 mg   d) 30 mg

2. A vial contains 1 mg of a drug in every 4 mL of solution. How many mL need to be drawn up for a dose of:
    a) 750 mcg   b) 500 mcg   c) 250 mcg   d) 100 mcg

3. A solution contains 2.5 mcg of a drug per 10 mL. How many mL need to be drawn up for a dose of:
    a) 1.25 mcg   b) 500 mcg   c) 625 mcg   d) 0.25 mcg

4. A bottle of medication contains 1 mg per 10 mL. How many mL are drawn into the syringe for a dose of:
    a) 2 mg   b) 1.5 mg   c) 0.1 mg   d) 500 mcg

Infusions, the giving set and infusion (or drip) rates

In this section a further factor is introduced into drug dosage calculations, that of *time*. Some fluids have to be *infused* into the body slowly over several hours.

Key point: Although infusion pumps are used to deliver intravenous fluids in many hospitals and other facilities, and it is easy to set a volume and rate, you will still need to be able to do the necessary calculations so that you know what numbers to insert.

The treatment sheet will indicate the amount of time required for the prescribed dose: for example, 1 litre over 8 hours. In most infusions a 'giving set' with a roller clamp is used to control the speed of the infusion; a drip chamber that delivers a pre-set volume of fluid per drop allows the nurse to see the drops and to set the drip rate. The drip rate is dependent on the volume to be infused, the time of the infusion and the size of each drop (sometimes called the 'drip factor').

Key point: in a standard giving set the volume of each drop is one-twentieth of a millilitre or 0.05 mL. This means that there are 20 drops in every 1 mL. In a burette giving set, there are 60 drops per millilitre.

The speed of the infusion, or drip rate, needs to be calculated in drops per minute.

Calculations involving drip rates usually require conversion from mL per hour to drops per minute.

The formula for calculating infusion rates is

$$\text{Rate (drops/min)} = \frac{\text{Volume of solution (mL)} \times \text{no. of drops/mL}}{\text{Time (minutes)}}$$

Example: 250 mL of fluid is to be given over two hours using a standard giving set (20 drops per mL). What is the infusion rate?

Step 1: convert to mL/hr.
Step 2: convert to drops/hr.
Step 3: convert to drops/minute.

Step 1: 250 mL in 2 hours = 250 ÷ 2 = 125 mL/hr.
Step 2: 125 × 20 = 2500 drops/hr.
Step 3: 2500 ÷ 60 cancels to 250 ÷ 6 then cancels to 125 ÷ 3.

$$\frac{41.67}{3\overline{)125.00}} = 42 \text{ drops per minute (to the nearest drop)}$$

Example: 1.5 litres is to be given over six hours using a burette (60 drops per mL) giving set. What is the correct rate for the infusion?

Step 1: 1.5 litres in 6 hours = 1500 ÷ 6 = 250 mL/hr.
Step 2: 250 × 60 = 15,000 drops/hr.
Step 3: 15,000 ÷ 60 = 250 drops/minute (to the nearest drop).

Test 45

1. Convert the following infusion rates to drops per minute.
   The giving set has 20 drops per mL.
   a) 200 mL in 40 minutes   b) 120 mL in 30 minutes
   c) 80 mL in 100 minutes   d) 90 mL in 1 hour

2. Convert the following infusion rates to drops per minute.
   The giving set has 20 drops per mL. Give your answers to the nearest drop.
   a) 200 mL/hr b) 250 mL/hr c) 500 mL in 6 hrs d) 1 L in 8 hrs

Concentration

The term *concentration* means the strength of the solution that contains the drug. By way of example, instant coffee is made by dissolving coffee power in hot water; you can make the drink (the *solution*) either strong or weak depending on the volume of water (the *diluent*) added and the quantity of coffee used. Two spoonfuls of coffee in 200 mL of water gives the same strength drink as one spoonful in 100 mL of water. Similarly, a vial containing 2 mg of a drug in 20 mL of solution has the same strength as a vial containing 1 mg of the same drug in 10 mL of solution. Different strengths are easily compared by considering how much drug is present in each 1 mL of solution (per mL; /mL).

Example: a vial contains 2.5 mg of a drug in 5 mL of solution. What is the concentration of the drug in mg per mL?

2.5 mg of drug are contained in 5 mL of solution so 1 mL must contain only one-fifth as much drug.
2.5 mg is contained in 5 mL so 1 mL contains 2.5 ÷ 5 = 0.5 mg per mL or 0.5 mg/mL.

The concentration is 0.5 mg/mL (0.5 mg of drug in every 1 mL). Concentrations can also be used to work out the quantity of drug in a given volume of solution.

Example: the concentration of a drug is 0.5 mg/mL. How many milligrams of drug are there in 1 litre?

First step: 1 litre = 1000 mL.
Second step: 0.5 mg in 1 mL and we have 1000 mL.
So milligrams of drug = 0.5 × 1000 = 500 mg.

Example: the concentration of a drug is 250 milligram/mL. How many grams are there in 100 mL?

First step: 250 mg = 250 ÷ 1000 g = 0.25 g.
Second step: 0.25 g in 1 mL and we have 100 mL.
So grams of drug = 0.25 × 100 = 25 g (25 g/100 mL).

Key point: the concentration of infusion fluids is usually measured in terms of percentage weight-volume (% w/v), where the weight (w) is in grams and the volume (v) is 100 mL.

So 1% w/v means 1 g per 100 mL of solution, 2% w/v means 2 g per 100 mL of solution etc.

'Sodium chloride 0.9 % w/v infusion fluid' has 0.9 g of sodium chloride dissolved in 100 mL of water.

Example: a 1 litre bag of saline (sodium chloride solution) is labelled as 0.9% w/v. How many grams of sodium chloride are there in the bag?

First step: 0.9 % w/v means 0.9 g per 100 mL (0.9 g/100 mL).
Second step: 1 litre = 1000 mL = 10 x100 mL.
= 10 × 0.9 g = 9 g.

Example: a 5 mL vial contains a drug at a strength of 0.1% w/v. How many milligrams are there in 1 mL of solution?

First step: 0.1% w/v means 0.1 g/100 mL.
Second step: convert 0.1 g to mg.
0.1 g = 0.1 × 1000 mg = 100 mg
So we have 100 mg/100 mL or 1 mg/1 mL (1 mg/mL).

From the above answer we can see that:

1 mg/mL = 0.1% w/v; 2 mg/mL = 0.2% w/v;
10 mg/mL = 1% w/v; 50 mg/mL = 5% w/v, etc.

Bags of saline labelled as 0.9% w/v contain sodium chloride at a concentration of 9 mg/mL, which is similar to that of blood plasma, making it safe to infuse and is known as *physiological saline* ('normal saline').

Key point: if you come across percentage weight-weight (% w/w), it means that both the drug and the diluent are measured by weight. In this case 1% w/w means 1 g per 100 g.

Test 46

Complete the following concentration items. They do not require any knowledge of drugs.

1. You have lignocaine hydrochloride for injection, 50 mg in 5 mL ampoules. What is the concentration in mg/mL?
2. You have lignocaine hydrochloride for injection, 100 mg in 5 mL ampoules. What is the concentration in mg/mL?
3. A PCA syringe contains 60 mg of morphine sulphate in 30 mL sodium chloride. What is the concentration of morphine in mg/mL?
4. 500 mg of amoxycillin sodium is dissolved in 12.5 mL of water. What is the concentration in mg/mL?
5. 1 g of amoxycillin sodium is dissolved in 20 mL of water. What is the concentration in mg/mL?
6. How many grams of glucose are there in a 500 mL bag of 5% w/v glucose in water for infusion ?
7. The patient is to receive an intravenous infusion of sodium chloride (0.18% w/v) and glucose (4% w/v). How much glucose is present in a 500 mL bag?
8. Zinc and castor oil cream contains 7.5% w/w zinc oxide. How much zinc oxide is present in a 25 g tube?
9. Danaparoid sodium contains 1250 units/mL. How many units are there in a 0.6 mL ampoule?
10. 10 mL of sterile Water for Injection BP is added to a vial containing 500 mg of vancomycin. What is a) the concentration of the reconstituted drug in mg/mL? and b) the approximate concentration of the infusion fluid in mg/mL if the 10 mL of solution is added to 250 mL of 5% glucose?

Higher-level calculations

These are longer questions that require additional steps to arrive at the answer. The key to answering these questions is to break them down into manageable chunks. This is done by making the more obvious calculations first, often starting with the information contained in the first sentence.

In the example below, the dose required is *proportional* to the patient's weight. So, for example, a patient weighing 100 kg will require twice the dose of a patient weighing 50 kg.

The *dose* is given in milligrams per kilogram (of body weight) per hour (mg/kg/hr).

The *infusion* rate is given in millilitres per hour (mL/hr).

The *drip* rate is given in drops per minute (drops/min).

Example: the treatment sheet indicates that you need to administer 1 g of a drug at a rate of 10 mg/kg/hr. The bag contains 1 g in 100 mL. If the patient weighs 80 kg, then:
  a) what is the drip rate using a standard giving set that delivers 20 drops per mL?
  b) how long should the infusion last?

The question looks complicated but is easily broken down into manageable chunks as follows:

a) Step 1:   The patient needs 10 mg per kg per hour
             = 10 × 80 mg per hour
             = 800 mg/hr (the dose prescribed per hour).

   Step 2:   Work out the volume of drug required per hour.
             No of mL = Dose prescribed ÷ Dose per bag × Volume of vial
             = (800 ÷ 200) × Volume of vial
             = 0.8 × 100
             = 80 mL/hr.

   Step 3:   Work out the number of drops for a standard giving set.
             80 mL × 20 drops = 1600 drops per hour

   Step 4:   Work out the drip rate in drops per minute.
             = 1600 ÷ 60
             = 80 ÷ 3
             = 27 drops/minute to the nearest drop.

b) To work out the length of the infusion we return to Step 2. The rate of the infusion is 800 mg/hr and we have to administer 1g (1000 mg). The time of the infusion is given by:
$^{1000}/_{800}$ hrs = $^{10}/_{8}$ = $^{5}/_{4}$ = $1^{1}/_{4}$ hours
(Check: 800 mg/hr × 1.25 hr = 1000 mg.)

Test 47

1. The treatment is a continuous intravenous infusion of dopamine. You have 400 mg of the drug, ready-mixed in 250 mL of 5% glucose infusion fluid. The rate of the infusion is to be 3 microgram/kg/minute and the patient weighs 89 kg. Calculate:
   a) the concentration of dopamine in the infusion fluid, in mg/mL
   b) the rate in micrograms/minute
   c) the rate in milligrams/minute
   d) the rate in milligrams/hour (to 1 decimal place)
   e) the rate in mL/hour (refer to your answer in a).
2. The prescription requires 40 microgram/kg/hr of diclofenac sodium to be given by an intravenous infusion.
   The stock is a 3 mL 25 mg/mL ampoule to be diluted to 500 mL with infusion fluid. If the patient weighs 75 kg calculate:
   a) the number of milligrams of diclofenac in one 500 mL bag;
   b) the rate in micrograms/hour;
   c) the rate in mg/hour;
   d) the concentration of diclofenac in the infusion fluid in mg/mL;
   e) the infusion rate in mL/hour;
   f) how many hours the infusion fluid will last.
3. The patient is prescribed gentamicin 80 mg to be infused over 30 minutes in a burette made up to 100 mL of 0.9% w/v sodium chloride. You have 2 mL ampoules containing 40 mg/mL. Calculate the infusion rate in drops per minute.

4. Lignocaine hydrochloride is to be given by intravenous infusion at a rate of 4 mg/minute. Stock is 0.2% w/v lignocaine in 5% w/v glucose infusion fluid. What is the infusion rate in mL/hour?

5. A patient weighing 100 kg is to receive an intravenous infusion of amiodarone 5 mg/kg over 2 hours. Stock is 3 mL ampoules containing 50 mg/mL and the diluent is 250 mL of 5% w/v glucose. Calculate:
   a) the number of milligrams of amiodarone to be administered
   b) the volume of amiodarone to be drawn up in millilitres
   c) the number of whole ampoules required to do this (round up)
   d) the total volume of fluid to be infused
   e) the rate of infusion rate in mL/hour using a burette that delivers 60 drops per mL.

6. A patient weighing 100 kg requires an intravenous infusion of sodium nitroprusside 1.5 micrograms/kg/minute given in 1 L of 5% glucose solution for 3 hours. The stock is a 10 mg/mL 5 mL vial. Calculate:
   a) the number of milligrams of drug to infuse
   b) the volume of drug to be drawn up from the 5 mL vial.

7. The treatment is acetylcysteine 50 mg/kg diluted in 500 mL of 5% glucose, for infusion over 4 hours. The drug comes in 10 mL ampoules of concentration 200 mg/mL. For a patient weighing 85 kg, calculate:
   a) the number of grams of acetylcysteine to infuse
   b) the exact number of ampoules required
   c) the total volume of solution to infuse
   d) the infusion rate in mL/minute to one decimal place.

8. You are to administer a continuous intravenous infusion of dobutamine hydrochloride 5 microgram/kg/minute to a patient weighing 83 kg. Stock is a 20 mL ampoule containing 125 mg of dobutamine. The entire contents are diluted with sodium chloride 0.9% w/v infusion fluid. How long will the solution last, to the nearest hour?

Changing the infusion rate

Some questions will ask you to work out a new infusion time or a new infusion rate, where the speed of an infusion is altered partway through. The key is to break the question into two parts. First, you have to work out the volume given before the infusion was stopped; and then the volume left to give when the infusion is restarted (and the time left to give it where the new rate is to be calculated).

Example: a 1 L bag of 0.9% saline is infused at a rate of 125 mL/hr for the first 6 hours and then increased to 150 mL/hr until the bag is finished. How long will the infusion last?

1) 125 mL/hr for 6 hours = 6 × 125 = 750 mL
2) Remainder = 1000 mL − 750 mL = 250 mL
Total time = 7 hr 40 min

Example: a 1 L bag of 0.9% saline is infused at a rate of 150 mL/hr for the first 4 hours. The rate is then decreased so that the infusion is complete after a further 4 hours. Calculate the new infusion rate in mL/hr.

1) 150 mL/hr for 4 hours = 4 × 150 = 600 mL
2) Remainder = 400 mL
400 mL ÷ 4 hr = 100 mL/hr

Test 48

1. An infusion of 1 litre of 0.9% saline is required. The pump is switched on at 08:30 hours and the flow rate is 100 mL/hour. After 4 hours the pump speed is reduced to 60 mL/hr. At what time will the infusion be complete?
2. A 1.5 L bottle of liquid is PEG tube fed via a pump. The rate is set to 125 mL/hr and the pump is switched on at 20:00 hours. The rate is increased at 06:00 hours. If the feed has finished by 07:00 hours, what was the rate increased to?

Calculating the prescribed dose in infusions

If you know the concentration of the drug and the speed of the pump it is possible to work 'backwards' to find the prescribed dose in, for example, mg/minute or microgram/kg/minute.

Example: a syringe pump containing 250 mg of frusemide in 250 mL of 0.9% sodium chloride is running at 48 mL/hr. What is the dose in mg/minute?

Step 1: The concentration in mg/mL: 250 mg ÷ 250 mL = 1 mg/mL.

Step 2: Convert the speed from mL/hr to mL/min:
48 mL/hr ÷ 60 min/hr = mL/min = 0.8 mL/min.

Take one minute: volume = 0.8 mL (step 2) and then the dose is: 0.8 mL × 1 mg/mL (in step 1) = 8 mg in one minute or 8 mg/min.

Example: a syringe pump contains 25 mg of dobutamine in 50 mL of 5% glucose solution. The pump is running at a speed of 72 mL/hr. What is the dose in micrograms/kg/minute for an 80 kg patient?

Step 1: Work out the concentration in micrograms/mL:
25 mg ÷ 50 mL = 0.5 mg/mL = 500 micrograms/mL.

Step 2: Work out the concentration in micrograms/kg/mL.
500 micrograms/mL ÷ 80 kg = 50 ÷ 8 = 6.25 micrograms/ kg/mL.

Step 3: Convert the speed from mL/hr to mL/min:
72 mL/hr ÷ 60 min/hr = 6/5 = 1.2 mL/min.

Take one minute: volume = 1.2 mL (step 3) and the dose is then: 6.25 microgram/kg × 1.2 mL (in step 2) = 7.5 microgram/kg in one minute or 7.5 microgram/kg/min.

Test 49

1. Calculate the dose of dobutamine in microgram/kg/minute for the following pump rates and patient body weights. The concentration of dobutamine in the syringe is 500 microgram/mL.

a) pump rate: 7.2 mL/hr; body weight: 60 kg
b) pump rate: 5.4 mL/hr; body weight: 90 kg
c) pump rate: 30 mL/hr; body weight: 100 kg
d) pump rate: 75 mL/hr body weight: 50 kg.

Chapter 4 questions

1. The prescription asks for bumetanide 4 mg. Stock is 1 mg tablets. How many do you give?
2. An ampoule contains frusemide 10 mg/mL. How much do you draw up for a dose of 20 mg?
3. The patient is prescribed 30 mg of metoclopramide by intramuscular injection. Stock is 5 mg/mL in 2 mL ampoules. How many ampoules are required?
4. The patient has been prescribed ranitidine 150 mg. Stock is ranitidine syrup, 75 mg/5 mL. How much do you give?
5. What volume of amitriptyline 25 mg/5 mL oral solution is required to give a dose of 75 mg?
6. You are to administer 5 mg of morphine sulphate by intramuscular injection. Stock ampoules contain 10 mg in 2 mL. How much do you give?
7. Erythromycin is prescribed for intravenous injection via a burette. 1 g of powder is reconstituted with Water for Injection BP to give 20 mL of solution. What volume of the solution should be added to the burette for a dose of 900 mg?
8. 100 mL of pre-mixed ciprofloxacin lactate contains 200 mg of the drug. How much do you give if the treatment sheet asks for 750 mg?
9. The patient needs 120 mg of procainamide by intravenous injection. If it is given at a rate of 30 mg/minute how long will the injection take?
10. If an infusion pump delivers 40 mL in 30 minutes, what is the infusion rate in mL/hour?
11. 30 mg of midazolam is to be infused over 12 hours in 1 L 0.9% normal saline using a burette. What is the infusion rate in mg/hour?

12. Quinine dihydrochloride 6% 20 mg/kg is infused over 4 hours. What is the dose per hour for a patient weighing 74 kg?

13. Ketamine is to be given by intramuscular injection. The dose is 10 mg/kg and the stock is a 100 mg/mL 10 mL vial. How much do you draw up for a patient weighing 82 kg?

14. Your patient has been written up for an intravenous infusion of terbutaline. A 500 micrograms/mL 5 mL ampoule is diluted with glucose 5% to a concentration of 10 micrograms/mL for infusion over 10 hours. What is the infusion rate in mL/hour?

15. Aciclovir 5% w/w cream is prescribed. How much aciclovir is present in a 2 g tube of cream?

16. One litre of physiological saline (0.9% w/v) is to be given over 6 hours with a 20 drop per mL giving set. What is the infusion rate in drops per minute (to the nearest drop)?

17. 1 g of amoxycillin is reconstituted with Water for Injection BP to give 20 mL of solution. What is the concentration of the drug in mg/mL?

18. 500 mg of amoxycillin powder is reconstituted with 2.5 mL of Water for Injection BP and then diluted to 50 mL with 0.9% sodium chloride infusion fluid. What is the concentration of the drug in mg/mL?

19. A 2.5 g dose of flucytosine is administered over 30 minutes by intravenous infusion. Stock is a 10 mg/mL infusion bottle. What is the volume infused?

20. A syringe pump containing 250 mg of frusemide in 125 mL of Hartmann's solution is running at a speed of 90 mL/hr. What is the dose in mg/minute?

5 Drug administration

In 2006, the Australian Health Ministers endorsed the recommendation made by the Australian Council for Safety and Quality in Health Care that a common in-patient medication chart be used in all public hospitals to assist in standardisation and consistent documentation of medications and their administration. The National In-Patient Medication Chart (NIMC) has been used in the examples in this chapter to help you to familiarise yourself with its format.

At this time in New Zealand, the Safe Medication Management (SMM) Program is developing medication chart standards for New Zealand hospitals. An example chart that meets these standards will be drafted (www.safemedication.org.nz, october 2008).

How to read medication charts

The introduction of a National In-patient Medication Chart (NIMC) is considered to be a significant quality improvement strategy aimed at addressing safety and quality issues associated with prescription, supply and administration of medications in hospitals.

The chart is intended to reflect best practice and assist clinicians in all steps of the medication management cycle for safer prescribing, dispensing and administration of medications in order to minimise the risk of adverse medication administration events. The first page of the NIMC is used for once only, pre-medication (i.e. before surgery) and nurse initiated medicines. For once-only and pre-medication orders the following must be documented in the correct columns: date prescribed, generic name of medication, route of administration (using the accepted abbreviation), dosage, date and time for administration, prescribers' signature and printed name, initials of the person administering the medication, the time and whether the drug is supplied (S) or is on imprest (I).

Nurse initiated medications applies to a limited list of medicines that hospital policy guidelines permit nurses to administer. Typically, this list includes simple analgesics (e.g. paracetamol), aperients (e.g. Agarol), antacids (e.g. Mylanta), cough suppressants, sublingual nitrates (e.g. Anginine), inhaled bronchodilators (e.g. Ventolin), artificial tear solution, sodium chloride 0.9% flush or infusion to maintain patency of intravenous lines. It is the nurse's responsibility to ensure that she or he knows, understands and abides by the government or hospital policy on nurse initiated medicines.

Telephone orders should be discouraged unless essential (e.g. rural areas, no on-site medical staff) in which case two nurses should independently receive the order and read it back to the prescribing medical officer. The following must be documented in the correct columns: date prescribed, generic name of medication, route of administration (using the correct abbreviation), dosage, date, time and frequency to be administered, the initials of the nurses confirming and checking the verbal order, the name of the medical officer giving the verbal order, and the record of administration.

Up to four doses can be administered and all telephone orders must be signed or otherwise confirmed in writing within 24 hours.

The second and third pages refer to regular medications and include specific sections for variable dose medications and anti-coagulants. The variable dose section is for those medications that require dosages based on laboratory test results (e.g. lithium carbonate) or as a reducing protocol (e.g. steroids). For each day of therapy the drug level test result and time of the test must be documented, along with the dosage, prescriber's initials, actual time of administration, and the initials of the administering nurse. The warfarin (anticoagulant) section is highlighted in red as an extra alert that it is a high-risk medicine. Almost 10% of the adult population now takes warfarin and it is regularly a drug that causes adverse events. It is recommended that clinicians consult the Guidelines for Anticoagulation using Warfarin (2003) available at www.health.vic.gov.au/vmac/downloads/warfarin_guidelines.pdf.

For each day of treatment, the following information should be documented: INR (International Normalised Ratio) result, dose of warfarin, prescriber's initials, and the initials of the two nurses checking and administering the dose. A standard dose time of 1600 hours (4pm) is recommended as this allows the medical officer to order the next dose based on the INR result. There is also provision on the NIMC for the nurse or medical officer to record that the patient has received counselling about the use of warfarin as well as written information.

An online module for the NIMC is now available from the National Prescribing Service:
Australian Council for Safety and Quality in Health Care
http//nimc.nps.org.au

The medication chart is a legal document and therefore must be written clearly, legibly and unambiguously. Every nurse has a responsibility to ensure that she or he can clearly read and understand an order before administering any medications. Where an order is unclear or incomplete, a medical officer must be contacted for clarification.

Never make any assumptions or jump to any conclusions about the prescriber's intent. If there is insufficient space on the chart to sign for the administration of medications, a new chart should be written as the medication orders should not be considered valid or current prescriptions.

Every medication chart must have the patient's identification details, either a current patient identification label or the same information printed legibly in black pen. The first prescriber is to print the patient's name and sign that the label is correct. If a patient has a known or suspected drug allergy or adverse drug reaction (ADR), these details must be completed in the section on the medication chart and signed. If there is no known allergy or reaction, the 'Nil Known' or 'Unknown' boxes are ticked.

No erasures or obliterations (e.g. with 'white out') can be used. Errors must be struck through and initialled. When a medication is not given, the nurse must record the reason for non-administration by entering the appropriate code in a circle and initialling the entry. If medications are withheld, the reason must be documented in the patient's hospital notes as well as on the medication chart.

It is appropriate to withhold a medication if there is a known adverse drug reaction (ADR) which must be documented on the chart. Generally medications should NOT be withheld if the patient is on Nil By Mouth (NBM) or fasting unless specifically requested by the medical officer. If a medication is not available on the ward, it is the nurse's responsibility to contact the pharmacy or medical officer in order to obtain a supply.

Because some drug dosages are dependent on a patient's weight or height, these must be recorded on the medication chart.

Finally, every nurse must observe **the five Rs** of medication administration: the **right** drug, the **right** dose, the **right** route, the **right** time and the **right** patient.

Abbreviations

Instructions for the administration of drugs are best written out in full in English without abbreviation. However, a lack of space on drug charts means that some abbreviations find widespread use. Most are easily understood except for a few in Latin that need to be remembered.

The following abbreviations may be used in some texts and you will see them on patients' medication charts. The following abbreviations have been deemed acceptable by the Australian Council for Safety and Quality in Health Care as at November 2008:

Route

Gutt = eye drop
IM = intramuscular injection
inh or INH = inhaled
IT = intrathecal
IV = intravenous injection
MDI = metered dose inhaler
NEB = nebulised
NG = via nasogastric tube
Occ = eye ointment
PCA = patient controlled analgesia
PEG = via percutaneous enteral gastrostomy
PO = orally, by mouth
PR = into the rectum
PV = into the vagina
subcut = subcutaneous injection
subling = under the tongue
top or TOP = topically

Measure and concentration

g = gram
L = litre
mcg = microgram (safer to write microgram in full)
mEq = milliequivalent
mg = milligram
mL = millilitre
mmol = millimole
Unit(s) = International Units

Doses must be written using metric and Arabic (e.g. 1, 2, 3, etc.) systems. **Never** use Roman numerals (i, ii, iii, iv, etc.). Always use zero (0.) before a decimal point (e.g. 0.5 mg) otherwise the decimal point may be missed. Never use a terminal zero (.0) as it may be misread if the decimal point is missed. Where possible, state or write the dose in whole numbers.

Frequency of administration

ac = before meals
bd = twice daily
mane = in the morning
nocte = at night
od (OD) = once daily
pc = after meals
prn = when required
qid = four times daily
stat = at once
tds = three times daily

The NIMC suggests administration times to coincide with these abbreviations.

The above lists are neither exclusive nor exhaustive and some health care facilities might use variations of these. However, many abbreviations have been considered dangerous by the Australian Council for Safety and Quality in Health Care because they are easily confused with others. It is your responsibility to know the abbreviations that are approved and accepted by your organisation and to use these consistently and correctly.

Prescription awareness

As a nurse you will encounter drugs and drug administration situations with which you are not familiar. Most difficulties can be solved by referring to an up-to-date issue of the MIMS handbook or MIMS Annual, or by consulting another registered nurse or a medical officer. The following questions and answers will help address some of the more common dilemmas that arise.

1. The patient is prescribed morphine sulphate 10–20 mg for post-operative analgesia. The patient is complaining of pain and you administer two 5 mL ampoules each containing 10 mg of morphine sulphate. Correct or incorrect?

Incorrect: start with the lowest dose, after assessing the patient's pain.

2. The patient is prescribed paracetamol 0.5–1 g every 4 to 6 hours prn to a maximum of 4 g daily. You give the patient 1 g at 0800 hrs. The patient requests a further dose at midday but you ask the patient to wait until 2 pm. Correct or incorrect?

Incorrect: the dose can be given every four hours at the patient's request (to a maximum of 4 g daily).

3. The patient is prescribed aspirin for pain relief. You have two strengths of tablet, 75 mg and 300 mg. You administer one 300 mg tablet. Correct or incorrect?

Correct: The standard dose is one 300 mg tablet when no dose is stated.

Test 50

1. A patient is prescribed warfarin 6 mg mane. Stock is 3 mg tablets. How many tablets will the patient receive in a two-day period?
2. The patient is prescribed sodium valproate 200 mg bd. How many milligrams will be given to the patient in a 24-hour period?
3. A patient is taking amoxycillin 500 mg tds. How many grams of amoxycillin will the patient consume in total if the treatment lasts five days?
4. The patient is written up for paracetamol 1 g qid. What is the total daily dose?
5. A patient is written up for frusemide 20 mg IM. How many 20 mg tablets will be given to the patient in 24 hours?

6. The prescription is 20 mL lactulose bd. How many full days supply of lactulose are there in a 500 mL bottle?
7. The patient is written up for haloperidol 0.5–1.5 gram mane or bd prn. What is the maximum daily dose?
8. The prescription states bisacodyl 5 mg po bd. How many milligrams of bisacodyl should the patient take each day?
9. The treatment is lansoprazole 30 mg mane for 8 weeks. Stock is 15 mg capsules. How many 30-capsule packs are required for the full treatment?
10. The patient is taking 2.5 mg of dexamethasone qid for 5 days. Stock tablets are 500 micrograms and 4 mg. How many dexamethasone tablets will be dispensed over the five-day period?
11. Morphine 5 mg IM every four hours is prescribed. How many milligrams is this daily?

Drug familiarity

The most time-consuming part of any drug round is finding the right medication in the drug trolley. This problem has eased with the use of patients' own drugs kept in bedside cabinets, often in blister packs. However, not all patients have their own drugs or a secure place to store them, so the ward drug trolley still finds widespread use. Finding medication improves quickly with practice, especially if the trolley is kept tidy, with the drugs arranged in alphabetical order.

The majority of drugs are prescribed by their approved (generic) name and not by the manufacturers' (brand) name. The brand name usually takes precedence on the packaging, with the approved name written in small print underneath. For this reason a good knowledge of brand names is an advantage in drug administration.

If a nurse informed you that she had given a patient two Panadol, what would this mean to you? Would you need to refer to the MIMS handbook to find out she meant one gram of paracetamol?.

Many patients have little knowledge about their medications. A patient who is prescribed the analgesic Di-Gesic for example, might not know it contains paracetamol. However, you should have a basic idea of a drug's purpose (indication) before administering it: for example analgesic, anti-emetic, anti-hypertensive, anti-depressant, antibiotic. This information is beyond the scope of this book but is available in the MIMS handbook.

Examples of some common medications and their brand names are shown in Table 5.1. You will find a list like this helpful in locating patients' medications in the drug trolley. Convention dictates that the generic name of a drug begins with a lower case letter, while the trade name takes an upper case letter. Some of the drugs have more than one brand name but only one name has been included in the list. Read through it carefully and slowly, then complete the test.

Table 5.1 Approved and brand names of common drugs

Approved name	Brand name	Approved name	Brand name	Approved name	Brand name
acetylcysteine	Parvolex	disulfiram	Antabuse	Ondansetron	Zofran
aciclovir	Zovirax	donepezil	Aricept	omeprazole	Losec
alendronate	Fosamax	domperidone	Motilium	pancrelipase	Creon
amisulpride	Solian	enoxaparin	Clexane	pantoprazole	Somac
atorvastatin	Lipitor	etanercept	Enbrel	paroxetine	Aropax
baclofen	Lioresal	etoricoxib	Arcoxia	potassium chloride	Slow-K
beclomethasone	Becotide	fluoxetine	Prozac	pramipexole	Sifrol
betahistine	Serc	frusemide	Lasix	perindopril	Coversyl
bisoprolol	Biocor	haloperidol	Serenace	prochlorperazine	Stemetil
budesonide	Pulmicort	hydrocortisone	Solu-Cortef	quetiapine	Seroquel
carbamazepine	Tegretol	hyoscine butylbromide	Buscopan	ranitidine	Zantac
ceftriaxone	Rocephin	ibuprofen	Brufen	risedronate	Actonel
chlorpromazine	Largactil	insulin glargine	Lantus	rivastigmine	Exelon
ciprofloxacin	Ciproxin	ipratropium bromide	Atrovent	ropinirole	Repreve
citalopram	Cipramil	lansoprazole	Zoton	rosiglitazone	Avandia
clarithromycin	Klacid	lercanidipine	Zanidip	salbutamol	Ventolin
clopidogrel	Plavix	meloxicam	Mobic	salmeterol	Serevent
carbidopa-levodopa	Sinemet	metoclopramide	Maxolon	senna	Senokot
danaparoid	Orgaran	metronidazole	Flagyl	silver sulfadiazine	Silvazine
darbepoetin alfa	Aranesp	midazolam	Hypnovel	sodium valproate	Epilim
diazepam	Valium	mirtazapine	Mirtazon	tamsulosin	Flomaxtra
diclofenac	Voltaren	nicorandil	Ikorel	tiotropium bromide	Spiriva
dipyridamole	Persantin	naloxone	Narcan	tolterodine tartrate	Detrusitol
				zopiclone	ImovaneT

Test 51

Check your knowledge of brand names by choosing the correct brand from A, B or C for the generic name shown.

	Generic	Brand A, B or C?	Answer
1.	ibuprofen	A. Panadol B. Brufen C. Di-Gesic	
2.	ciprofloxacin	A. Ciproxin B. Cipramil C. Clinoril	
3.	citalopram	A. Molipaxin B. Caprilon C. Cipramil	
4.	aciclovir	A. Zovirax B. Zanidip C. Zantac	
5.	metronidazole	A. Nysran B. Flagyl C. Zovirax	
6.	insulin glargine	A. Mixtard B. Humulin C. Lantus	
7.	enoxaparin	A. Clexane B. Orgaran C. Hepsal	

	Generic	Brand A, B or C?	Answer
8.	isorbide mononitrate	A. Monomax B. Flomax C. Lasix	
9.	lansoprazole	A. Losec B. Protium C. Zoton	
10.	cyclizine	A. Serc B. Valoid C. Buscopan	
11.	diclofenac	A. Voltaren B. Aricept C. Nozinan	
12.	valproate	A. Epilim B. Creon C. Enbrel	
13.	ranitidine	A. Zanidip B. Losec C. Zantac	
14.	metoclopramide	A. Valoid B. Persantin C. Maxolon	
15.	budenoside	A. Ventolin B. Serevent C. Symbicort	
16.	perindopril	A. Actonel B. Coversyl C. Ikorel	

	Generic	Brand A, B or C?	Answer
17.	carbamazepine	A. Tegretol B. Detrusitol C. Exelon	
18.	bisoprolol	A. Bicor B. Sinemet C. Xatral	
19.	clopidrogel	A. Lasix B. Plavix C. Pabrinex	
20.	ondansetron	A. Stemetil B. Maxalon C. Zofran	

Test 52

Refer to the container labels on the next two pages to answer the following questions.

1. The order is for an intravenous infusion of ciprofloxacin 400 mg bd given over 1 hour. What is the infusion rate in mL/hour?
2. The patient takes 30 mg of baclofen daily in three divided doses. How many 5 mL spoonfuls will you administer per dose?
3. An injection of enoxaparin is required. The dose is 0.5 mg per kg and the patient weighs 60 kg. What volume of enoxaparin must be expelled from the pre-filled syringe 100 mg/mL before the injection can be given?
4. The treatment is an intravenous infusion of imipenem with cilastatin. 1.5 g is to be given daily in three divided doses. How many vials will be needed each day?
5. The patient needs a 10 mg bolus dose of metoclopramide to be given by slow intravenous injection. How much should you draw up?
6. The client takes 20 mg of fluoxetine each day. Exactly what amount should you measure out?
7. The treatment sheet shows that 'four 5 mL spoonfuls of carbamazepine' are to be administered. How many milligrams of the drug is this?
8. The treatment sheet reads glyceryl trinitrate 400 mcg s/l prn. What does the patient need to take?

Clexane® Syringes

enoxaparin sodium

Solution for Injection

10 x **0.4** ml Pre-filled syringes   ✯*Aventis*

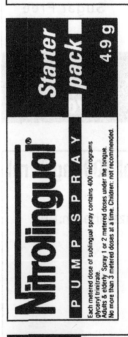

Starter pack 4.9 g

Nitrolingual® PUMP SPRAY

Each metered dose of sublingual spray contains 400 micrograms glyceryl trinitrate.
Adults & elderly Spray 1 or 2 metered doses under the tongue.
No more than 3 metered doses at a time. Children: not recommended.

Lioresal 5 mg/5 ml Liquid

Baclofen Ph.Eur.

To be taken by mouth

Ciba   POM

500 mg   Monovial pack

PRIMAXIN® IV 500 mg
(imipenem/cilastatin sodium)
Powder for solution for infusion
For intravenous use
single vial pack

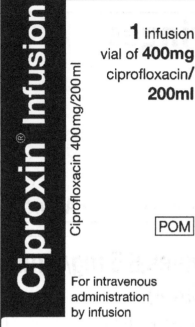

1 infusion
vial of **400mg**
ciprofloxacin/
200ml

POM

For intravenous
administration
by infusion

Bayer

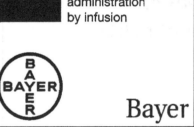

Metoclopramide
Injection

10 mg in 2 ml

10 ampoules each containing 2 ml
solution for i.m. or i.v. injection.

10 mg in 2 ml

≋ **hameln**
 pharmaceuticals

ESSENTIAL GENERICS

Fluoxetine

20 mg/5 ml

Oral Solution

Sugar Free

70 ml

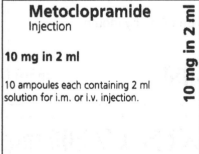

**Tegretol 100 mg/5 ml
Liquid**
Carbamazepine Ph.Eur.

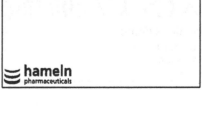

To be taken by mouth

Geigy   POM

Medication chart questions

This section tests your ability to read medication charts (treatment sheets). Study the charts carefully and answer the true/false items below. Provide a rationale for each response. In practice, how long you take to complete the drug round is far less important than the need to avoid making a mistake.

Example

Using the medication chart on page 98, decide whether the statements written below are true or false. The boxes with a nurse's signature inside show which nurse has administered the drug and at what time of day.

1 The patient's name is Steven Williams.

TRUE/FALSE

2. 15 mL of lactulose are to be administered in the morning and again in the evening.

TRUE/FALSE

3. You have atenolol 25 mg stock and should administer two tablets in the morning.

TRUE/FALSE

4. You should give the patient an injection of frusemide in the morning.

TRUE/FALSE

Explanation of answers

1. False, the given name is spelt differently (and in practice you should have checked it against the patient's arm band).
2. True, the right dose given at the right times.
3. True. This is the correct dose and time.
4. False, the correct route for administering the drug is orally. Moreover, the prescriber has not signed the chart.

Sample medication chart

Test 53

Using the medication chart shown on page 99, decide whether the statements below are true or false. Provide rationales for your responses.

1. The patient's name is Christopher Johns.

    TRUE/FALSE

2. The patient has been prescribed 4 g of paracetamol daily.

    TRUE/FALSE

3. The patient's next dose of omeprazole will be one 20 mg capsule, which is due on 6 July in the morning.

TRUE/FALSE

4. The patient's next dose of paracetamol is two 500 mg tablets to be given in the morning of 5 July.

TRUE/FALSE

5. The patient is written up for perindopril. The stock is 2 mg tablets. At 8 pm on 4 July you should have administered two 4 mg tablets.

TRUE/FALSE

Test 53 medication chart

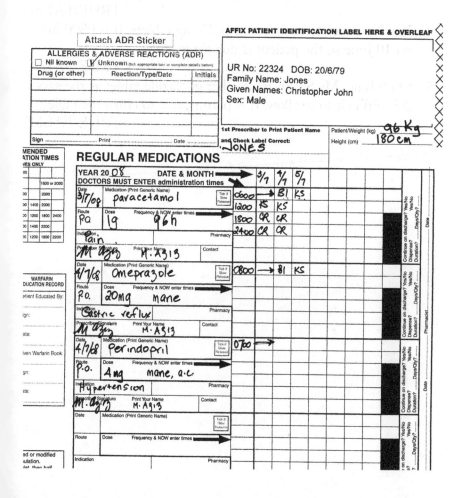

Test 54

Using the medication chart on page 101, decide whether the statements written below are true or false. Provide rationales for your responses.

1. The patient's name is Mary Smith.

   TRUE/FALSE

2. 25 mg milligram of thyroxine has been prescribed and it should be administered first thing in the morning.

   TRUE/FALSE

3. The patient is taking 150 mg of diclofenac per day.

   TRUE/FALSE

4. You have diclofenac in stock as 25 mg tablets. It is 0800 hrs on 10 June so the patient is due three tablets.

   TRUE/FALSE

5. On 9 June, Ms Smith refuses her gliclazide tablet as she says it is difficult to swallow. It is permissable to crush the table.

   TRUE/FALSE

Test 54 medication chart

Attach ADR Sticker

ALLERGIES & ADVERSE REACTIONS (ADR)

☑ Nil known   ☐ Unknown (tick appropriate box or complete details below)

Drug (or other)	Reaction/Type/Date	Initials

Sign .... Print .... Date ....

AFFIX PATIENT IDENTIFICATION LABEL HERE & OVERLEAF

UR No: 216201   DOB: 14/8/65
Family Name: Smith
Given Names: Mary
Sex: Female

1st Prescriber to Print Patient Name and Check Label Correct:
A. AHMED

Patient/Weight (kg) __76kg__
Height (cm) __167cm__

RECOMMENDED ADMINISTRATION TIMES — GUIDELINES ONLY

0800			
	1800 or 2000		
0800	2000		
0800	1400	2000	
0600	1200	1800	2400
0600	1400	2200	
0600	1200	1800	2200

WARFARIN EDUCATION RECORD

Patient Educated By:
Sign:
Date:
Given Warfarin Book:
Sign:
Date:

...ained or modified ...ormulation. ...tablet, then half ...ven.

REGULAR MEDICATIONS

YEAR 20 **08**   DATE & MONTH
DOCTORS MUST ENTER administration times

		5/6	6/6	7/6	8/6	9/6	10/6
Date 5/6/08 Medication (Print Generic Name) **thyroxine** Tick if Slow Release	0600	KS	CR	BI	IS	CR	CR
Route P.O. Dose 25mcg. Frequency & NOW enter times mane. a.c.							
Indication M xoedema Pharmacy							
Prescriber Signature A. Ahmed Print Your Name A. AHMED Contact							
Date 5/6/08 Medication (Print Generic Name) **diclofenac** Tick if Slow Release	0800	KS	CR	BI	KS	CR	CR
Route pa Dose 75mg Frequency & NOW enter times b.d.	2000	KS	CR	BI	KS	CR	
Indication Arthritis Pharmacy							
Prescriber Signature A. Ahmed Print Your Name A. AHMED Contact							
Date 5/6/08 Medication (Print Generic Name) **gliclazide** ☑ Tick if Slow Release	0800	KS	CR	BI	KS	℞	
Route PO. Dose 30mg Frequency & NOW enter times Mane							
Indication Diabetes Pharmacy							
Prescriber Signature A. Ahmed Print Your Name A. AHMED Contact							
Date Medication (Print Generic Name) Tick if Slow Release							
Route Dose Frequency & NOW enter times							
Indication Pharmacy							
Prescriber Signature Print Your Name Contact							

(right margin repeated for each medication block: Continue on discharge? Yes/No Dispense? Yes/No Duration? Days/Qty? Date / Pharmacist)

Test 55

Using the medication chart on page 103, decide whether the statements below are true or false. Provide rationales for your responses.

1. The patient's name is Lee Xiang.

   TRUE/FALSE

2. The nurse should give half a digoxin table on 3 July.

   TRUE/FALSE

3. The patient is to have her digitalis checked on 4 July.

   TRUE/FALSE

4. The warfarin dose varies from day to day. The next dose is 7 mg. Tablets come in strengths of 0.5, 1, 3 and 5 mg. The number of warfarin tablets to be administered on the evening of 3 July is two.

   TRUE/FALSE

5. The patient is unable to swallow the Slow-K tablets. It is permissable to crush them and mix them with jam.

   TRUE/FALSE

Test 55 medication chart

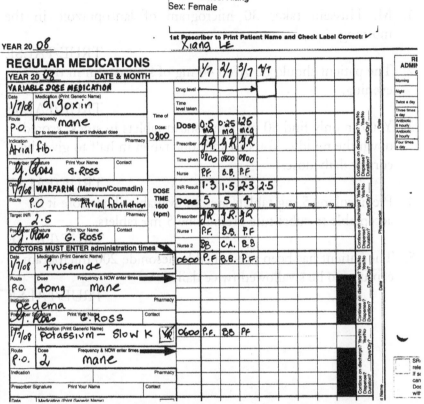

**AS REQUIRED
"PRN"
MEDICATIONS**

AFFIX PATIENT IDENTIFICATION LABEL HERE

UR No: 131909 DOB: 17/4/70
Family Name: Le
Given Names: Xiang
Sex: Female

1st Prescriber to Print Patient Name and Check Label Correct: ✓

YEAR 20 __08__

Xiang Le

REGULAR MEDICATIONS

YEAR 20 08 — DATE & MONTH: 1/7 | 2/7 | 3/7 | 4/7

VARIABLE DOSE MEDICATION

Date 1/7/08 Medication (Print Generic Name) **digoxin**
Route **P.O.** Frequency **mane**
Dr to enter dose time and individual dose
Indication **Atrial fib.**
Prescriber Signature **G. Ross** Print Your Name **G. ROSS** Contact

Drug level → ☐
Time level taken
Time of Dose: **0800**

Dose	0.5 mg	0.25 mg	125 mcg
Prescriber	GR	GR	GR
Time given	0800	0800	0800
Nurse	P.F.	B.B.	P.F.

WARFARIN (Marevan/Coumadin) 1/7/08
Route **P.O** Indication **Atrial fibrillation**
Target INR **2.5**
Prescriber Signature **G. Ross** Print Your Name **G. ROSS** Contact

DOSE TIME 1600 (4pm)

INR Result	1.3	1.5	2.3	2.5
Dose	5 mg	5 mg	4 mg	
Prescriber	GR	GR	GR	
Nurse 1	P.F.	B.B.	P.F	
Nurse 2	BB	C.A.	B.B	

DOCTORS MUST ENTER administration times ➤

Date 1/7/08 Medication (Print Generic Name) **frusemide**
Route **P.O.** Dose **40mg** Frequency & NOW enter times ➤ **mane**
Indication **oedema**
Prescriber Signature **G. Ross** Print Your Name **G. ROSS** Contact

0600	P.F.	B.B.	P.F.

Date 1/7/08 Medication (Print Generic Name) **potassium — Slow K** GR
Route **P.O.** Dose **2** Frequency & NOW enter times ➤ **mane**
Indication
Prescriber Signature Print Your Name Contact

0600	P.F.	BB	PF

Date Medication (Print Generic Name)

Test 56

Using the medication chart on page 105, decide whether the statements below are true or false. Provide rationales for your responses.

1. Mr Hussein takes 30 microgram of lansoprazole in the morning.

TRUE/FALSE

2. The patient should be given 40 mg of simvastatin in the evening.

TRUE/FALSE

3. You can only find 80 mg simvastatin tablets in stock, scored down the middle. You can split one tablet in half to give the correct daily dose.

TRUE/FALSE

4. Prednisolone 5 mg tablets are not available. Therefore it is acceptable to substitute prednisone 5 mg tablets.

TRUE/FALSE

5. The patient has been prescribed budesonide 200 microgram capsules to be swallowed twice daily.

TRUE/FALSE

Test 56 medication chart

AFFIX PATIENT IDENTIFICATION LABEL HERE & OVERLEAF

Attach ADR Sticker

ALLERGIES & ADVERSE REACTIONS (ADR)
☐ Nil known ☑ Unknown (tick appropriate box or complete details below)

Drug (or other)	Reaction/Type/Date	Initials

Sign .... Print .... Date ....

UR No: 331245   DOB: 4/12/44
Family Name: Hussein
Given Names: Mohammed Ali
Sex: Male

1st Prescriber to Print Patient Name and Check Label Correct: ✓
MOHAMMED HUSSEIN

Patient/Weight (kg) 105 Kg
Height (cm) 172 cm

RECOMMENDED ADMINISTRATION TIMES
LINES ONLY

0600			
	1800 or 2000		
0800	2000		
0600	1400	2000	
0600	1200	1800	2400
0600	1400	2200	
0600	1200	1800	2200

REGULAR MEDICATIONS

YEAR 20 **08**   **DATE & MONTH ➡**
DOCTORS MUST ENTER administration times ➡

	1/8	2/8	3/8					

Date 1/8/2008 **Medication (Print Generic Name)** lansoprazole ☐ Tick if Slow Release
Route PO **Dose** 30mg **Frequency & NOW enter times ➡** mane a.c.
0700 | TD | KS | CR
Indication reflux   **Pharmacy**
Prescriber Signature ⟋ **Print Your Name** J. SMITH   **Contact**

Date 1/8/08 **Medication (Print Generic Name)** simvastatin ☐ Tick if Slow Release
Route P.O **Dose** 40mg **Frequency & NOW enter times ➡** nocte
2000 | BP | BP | CR
Indication lipidaemia   **Pharmacy**
Prescriber Signature ⟋ **Print Your Name** J. SMITH   **Contact**

Date 1/8/08 **Medication (Print Generic Name)** prednisolone ☐ Tick if Slow Release
Route PO **Dose** 5mg **Frequency & NOW enter times ➡** daily
0800 | TD | KS | CR
Indication inflammation   **Pharmacy**
Prescriber Signature ⟋ **Print Your Name** JSMITH   **Contact**

Date 1/8/08 **Medication (Print Generic Name)** budesonide ☐ Tick if Slow Release
Route inh. **Dose** 200 mcg **Frequency & NOW enter times ➡** b.d.
0800 | TD | KS | CR.
1800 | BP | BP | CR
Indication   **Pharmacy**
Prescriber Signature **Print Your Name**   **Contact**

(right margin, repeated per row): Continue on discharge? Yes/No Dispensed? Days/City? Duration? Date / Pharmacist

WARFARIN EDUCATION RECORD

Patient Educated By:

Sign: ....

Date: ....

Given Warfarin Book:

Sign: ....

Date: ....

(bottom left, partial text): ...tained or modified ...ormulation. ...tablet, then half ...ven. ...st be swallowed

Test 57

Using the medication chart on page 107, decide whether the statements below are true or false. Provide rationales for your responses.

1. Mrs Luciano takes alendronate 70 mg once weekly in the morning before breakfast.

   TRUE/FALSE

2. The next dose of alendronate 70 mg is due on 18 October.

   TRUE/FALSE

3. There is no cephalexin 500 mg in stock so ceftriaxone can be substituted.

   TRUE/FALSE

4. The generic name for Di-Gesic must be written, not the trade name.

   TRUE/FALSE

Test 57 medication chart

Attach ADR Sticker			AFFIX PATIENT IDENTIFICATION LABEL HERE & OVERLEAF

ALLERGIES & ADVERSE REACTIONS (ADR)
- ☐ Nil known ☐ Unknown (tick appropriate box or complete details below)

Drug (or other)	Reaction/Type/Date	Initials
Penicillin	Rash	JB

Sign ...JBlack... Print J. BLACK Date 17/10/08

UR No: 53321 DOB: 25/11/47
Family Name: Luciano
Given Names: Maria Sophia
Sex: Female

1st Prescriber to Print Patient Name and Check Label Correct: ✓
MARIA LUCIANO

Patient/Weight (kg): 108 Kg
Height (cm): 162 cm

RECOMMENDED ADMINISTRATION TIMES — ROUTINES ONLY

0800		
	1800 or 2000	
0800	2000	
0800	1400	2000
0600	1200	1800	2400
0600	1400	2200
0600	1200	1800	2200

WARFARIN EDUCATION RECORD

Patient Educated By: ....
Sign: ....
Date: ....
Given Warfarin Book: ....
Sign: ....
Date: ....

...ained or modified ...ormulation. ...tablet, then half ...ven. ...t be swallowed ...ushing.

REGULAR MEDICATIONS

YEAR 20 08 DATE & MONTH ➡
DOCTORS MUST ENTER administration times ➡

			11/10	12/10	13/10	14/10	15/10	16/10	17/10	18/10
Date 17/10/08 **Medication (Print Generic Name)** alendronate ☐ Tick if Slow Release	**0700**	✕	KS						
Route P.O. **Dose** 70mg **Frequency & NOW enter times** Weekly a.c., mane									
Indication Osteoporosis **Pharmacy**									
Prescriber Signature JBlack **Print Your Name** J. BLACK **Contact**									
Date 11/10/08 **Medication (Print Generic Name)** cephalexin ☐ Tick if Slow Release	**0600**	JR	KS	MX					
Route po **Dose** 500mg **Frequency & NOW enter times** 96h.	**1200**	JR	KS						
	1800	PD	MX						
Indication U.T.I **Pharmacy**	**2400**	PD	MX						
Prescriber Signature JBlack **Print Your Name** J. BLACK **Contact**									
Date 16/10/08 **Medication (Print Generic Name)** DI-gesic ☐ Tick if Slow Release	**0800**								
Route po **Dose** 2 **Frequency & NOW enter times** tds	**1400**	➡ MX							
	2000	➡ MO							
Indication Pain **Pharmacy**									
Prescriber Signature JBlack **Print Your Name** J. BLACK **Contact**									
Date **Medication (Print Generic Name)** ☐ Tick if Slow Release									
Route **Dose** **Frequency & NOW enter times**									
Indication **Pharmacy**									
Prescriber Signature **Print Your Name** **Contact**									

Continue on discharge? Yes/No Dispense? Yes/No Days/Qty? .... Duration? .... Date ....

(Right column repeated vertical text): Continue on discharge? Yes/No Dispense? Yes/No Days/Qty? .... Duration? .... Pharmacist / Date / Name

6 Mock tests

Introduction to the tests

This final section contains a numeracy self-assessment test of 30 questions followed by three nursing calculation mock tests of 50 questions each. Each test comes with expanded answers (page 149). The numerical test is multiple choice: choose from answer A, B, C or D and circle it. To complete the three mock tests you will first have to decide what type of question is being asked and what calculations are necessary. There are four basic types of calculation, which are:

1. Unit conversion
2. Drug dosage
3. Concentrations
4. Rates

1. Make sure you are familiar with the metric system of measurement, especially metric weights and volumes and their abbreviations.
   Maths required: multiplication and division by powers of 10 (especially by 1000) and the positioning of the decimal point.
2. When calculating the amount of medication (number of tablets, ampoules, etc.) make sure that the dose prescribed and the dose to be administered are in the same metric units.

Maths required: division, multiplication and cancelling of fractions and whole numbers.

3. Concentrations can be used to work out the quantity of drug in a given volume of solution.

   Maths required: multiplication of whole numbers and decimals.

4. *Rate* questions always include the *time period*. Expect to have to work out either the length of time needed to administer a prescribed dose, or the total amount of drug infused for a given time period, or the *drip* rate.

   Maths required: multiplication and division of whole numbers, fractions and decimals.

Time limits have been set for the tests. The numerical test should be easy to complete in the allotted time. The three mock tests are more difficult. Only the best candidates will be able to complete all of the questions in the hour allowed. If you get stuck on a question, *you must leave it* and move on to the next question. Aim to pick up as many marks as you can as quickly as possible by answering the easier questions first. These are usually the shorter questions or 'one liners'. You get one mark for answering an easy question correctly and one mark for answering a difficult question correctly. Your goal is to achieve 100% accuracy as there is no room for error in drug calculations.

No special knowledge of drugs is required to answer the tests. Calculators should not be used to answer any of the questions.

Nursing numerical test

Time allowed: 30 minutes
NO CALCULATORS
Choose answer A, B, C or D and circle it.

1. How many hours are there between 07:00 hours and 16:30 hours?
    A 7.5 hours   B 8.5 hours   C 9.5 hours   D 10.5 hours

2. What is 400 mg in grams?
    A 0.25 g   B 0.4 g   C 0.25 g   D 0.04 g

3. A nursing test contains 40 questions. You answer 32 questions correctly. What is this in percent?
    A 70%   B 75%   C 80%   D 90%

4. What is 2200 mL in litres?
    A 22 L   B 2 L   C 0.2L   D 2.2L

5. If 15 is divided by 9 what is the answer to three decimal places?
    A 0.67   B 1.67   C 1.666   D 1.667

6. What is 25.4 ÷ 0.04?
    A 635   B 101.6   C 63.5   D 10.16

7. How many micrograms are there in 0.05 milligrams?
    A 0.5   B 5   C 50   D 500

8. One 0.1 mL drop of water drips from a tap every three seconds. How much water is wasted per hour?
    A 12 mL   B 120 mL   C 1.2 L   D 12 L

9. What is 200 milligrams as a fraction of 1 gram?
    A ¼   B ⅕   C ½   D ⅖

10. You have $4.50 and then spend 85 cents. How much money do you have left?
    A $3.55   B $3.45   C $3.75   D $3.65

11. What is the weight in kg when 10 g is added to 1 kg?
    A 1.001 kg   B 1.10 kg   C 1.01 kg   D 10.1 kg

12. A 500 mL bottle is three-quarters full of liquid. How much liquid does it contain?
    A 375 mL   B 360 mL   C 400 mL   D 350 mL

13. There are eight men and 42 women in a class of nursing students. What percentage are men?
    A 16%   B 24%   C 10%   D 12%

14. $25 \div \frac{5}{6} =$
    A 15   B 20   C 25   D 30

15. $\frac{5}{8}$ as a decimal is:
    A 0.625   B 0.675   C 0.725   D 0.75

16. $4(4 \times 3 - 2) =$
    A 46   B 40   C 14   D 16

17. $3\frac{3}{16} \times 1\frac{1}{3} =$
    A 4.25   B 4.5   C 5   D 5.25

18. 60 % as a fraction is:
    A $\frac{5}{6}$ B $\frac{3}{5}$ C $\frac{2}{3}$ D $\frac{7}{10}$

19. If your shift started at 07:30 hours and finished at 17:00 hours, how many hours were you on duty if you took a 30-minute lunch break?
    A 9 hours   B 8.5 hours   C 8.0 hours   D 7.5 hours

20. Dividing 20 by 0.004 gives:
    A 50   B 500   C 5000   D 50 000

21. Expressed as a decimal 22% is:
    A 0.11   B 0.22   C 2.2   D 0.2

22. If 1.8 gram of a drug is divided into four equal doses, how much is one dose?
    A 350 mg   B 375 mg   C 450 mg   D 475 mg

23. A 7 mg dose of a drug is prescribed. Tablets come in sizes of 1, 3, and 5 mg. What is the least number of tablets you can administer?

    A 7   B 5   C 4   D 3

24. A patient takes 500 mg of a drug every six hours. How many grams is this per day?

    A 2 g   B 3 g   C 4 g   D 5 g

25. A pump delivers 125 mL of fluid per hour. How long will it take to deliver one litre?

    A 9 hours   B 8 hours   C 7 hours   D 6 hours

26. 30 mg ÷ 12 =

    A 2.4 mg   B 2.5 mg   C 4 mg   D 0.25 mg

27. If a man weighing 90 kg loses 10% of his weight in hospital, what is his new weight?

    A 78   B 79g   C 80g   D 81g

28. Which of the fractions is the same size as five-sixths?

    A $^{16}/_{24}$ B $^{14}/_{18}$ C $^{25}/_{30}$ D $^{9}/_{12}$

29. What is 4% of 2 litres?

    A 8 mL   B 10 mL   C 40 mL   D 80 mL

30. 1 gram − 25 milligrams =

    A 0.975 g   B 907.5 mg   C 990.75 mg   D 1.975 mg

Nursing calculation mock test 1

Time allowed: one hour.
NO CALCULATORS

1. The patient takes 700 mg of allopurinol daily, divided into three doses. 200 mg is given at midday and again in the evening. What dose is given in the morning?
2. Convert 0.025 milligrams to micrograms.
3. The patient inhales 1.2 mg of budesonide powder daily. How many 200 microgram capsules is this?
4. Metformin is prescribed: 500 mg with breakfast for 10 days, followed by 500 mg with breakfast and evening meal for the next 10 days, then 500 mg with breakfast, lunch and evening meal for the next 10 days. How many grams of metformin has the patient taken in total in 30 days?
5. 40 mg of gliclazide is prescribed. Stock is 80 mg tablets scored. What do you give?
6. The prescription asks for carbamazepine 600 mg b.d. How many grams of carbamazepine does the patient take daily?
7. The patient is prescribed dexamethasone 2 mg q6h PO for 2 days. What is the total amount of dexamethasone taken over this period?
8. The patient needs 150 mg of amitriptyline. The stock is an oral solution containing 50 mg in 5 mL. What volume do you measure out?
9. An oral solution of verapamil contains 40 mg of the drug in 5 mL of solution. What is the concentration in mg/mL?
10. How many grams of dextrose are there in 20 mL of 5% w/v dextrose infusion fluid?
11. Change 200 micrograms/minute to mg/hour.
12. The treatment is 1 sachet of clarithromycin b.d. for 7 days. If each sachet contains 250 mg of clarithromycin to be reconstituted in 5mL water, how many grams of the drug in total will be consumed over the seven-day period?
13. The patient is written up for paracetamol 1g qid. If the tablets are 500 mg each, how many do you give per day?

14. 500 mL of dextrose 5% is administered at a rate of 100 mL/hour. How long will the infusion last?
15. The prescription reads gentamicin 160 mg stat IM. You have ampoules containing 40 mg/mL in 6 mL. What volume should you give?
16. An infusion pump is set to deliver 50 mL of infusion fluid per hour. The pump is switched on at 1100 hrs. How much should it have infused by 1330 hrs?
17. Metoclopramide oral solution is to be given. The dose is 10 mg and the stock strength is 5 mg in 5 mL. How much do you give?
18. The patient is given 0.5 millilitres of concentrated oral morphine solution 100 mg/5 mL. How many milligrams is this?
19. If 80 mg of pethidine is to be administered IM and the stock is a 50 mg/mL in 2 mL ampoules, what volume should be drawn up?
20. The patient needs naloxone by intravenous injection. Stock is a 400 microgram/mL. What volume do you draw up for a dose of 150 microgram? Give your answer to the nearest one hundredth of an mL (to two decimal points).
21. The patient has been prescribed hyoscine hydrobromide 0.6 mg SC every 4 hours. How many micrograms are there in one dose?
22. The prescription asks for alfacalcidol oral drops 2 micrograms/mL. If there are 20 drops per mL, how many micrograms are there in one drop?
23. Glycerine suppositories contain 70% w/w glycerol as active ingredient. How much glycerol is contained in one 4 gram suppository?
24. The patient is given 50 mL of 20% w/v glucose intravenously. How many grams of glucose is this?
25. The maximum daily dose of metoclopramide is 500 microgram/kg. How many milligrams of metoclopramide can a patient weighing 75 kg take every 24 hours?

26. Diazepam is diluted for infusion to give a solution containing 80 mg/L. If after 8 hours the patient had received 48 mg of diazepam what was the infusion rate in mL/hour?

27. An infusion of amiodarone is ordered to run at 0.5 mg/minute for 6 hours. How much amiodarone should be drawn up?

28. You are to administer 600 mg of dipyridamole per day in 3 divided doses of equal size. You have an oral suspension 50 mg per 5 mL. How much do you give per dose?

29. Heparin is to be given by subcutaneous injection. A 0.2 mL syringe of heparin contains 25,000 units of heparin per mL. How many units are there per syringe?

30. The treatment is an intravenous infusion of flecainide 100 microgram/kg/hour for 12 hours. The patient weighs 60 kg and the stock is 15 mL ampoules containing 10 mg/mL . What volume of flecainide will need to be drawn up and added to the infusion fluid?

31. The patient has been prescribed 1.5 mg of digoxin to be given in 4 divided doses of equal size, 6 hours apart. How many milligrams are there in one divided dose?

32. A 1.2 g vial of co-amoxiclav (Augmentin) powder is reconstituted to give 20 mL of solution. How much should be added to the infusion bag for a dose of 1 gram? Give your answer to the nearest tenth of a millilitre (to one decimal place).

33. The patient self-administers glyceryl trinitrate (GTN) aerosol spray, 400 microgram per metered dose. How many milligrams of GTN are contained in a 200-dose unit?

34. The prescription is disodium etidronate 5 mg/kg. You have 200 mg tablets and the patient weighs 80 kg. How many tablets are required?

35. A 5 mL ampoule of co-trimoxazole 96 mg/mL is diluted with glucose 5% w/v to give 125 mL of intravenous infusion fluid. If the patient receives a dose of 8 mg/minute, what is the infusion rate in mL/hour?

36. A fentanyl transdermal patch has been prescribed. It releases fentanyl through the skin at a rate of 100 microgram/hour for

three days. How much fentanyl will have been released after this time?

37. Cefuroxime is prescribed by intravenous infusion. 1 g of powder is reconstituted with 50 mL of 5% w/v glucose and the solution given over 40 minutes. How many milligrams per minute does the patient receive?

38. What is 1 mL/minute converted to litres/day?

39. Lignocaine 0.2% is available ready mixed in glucose 5% w/v infusion fluid. If the infusion rate is set at 4 mg/minute, what is the flow rate in mL/hour?

40. The patient is started on 0.9% w/v sodium chloride by subcutaneous infusion using a 20 drops/mL giving set. You check the drip rate and see that it is 14 drops in 30 seconds. Approximately what volume would you expect to see infused after 12 hours?

41. 500 mg of amoxicillin is reconstituted with 2.5 mL of water and then diluted with sodium chloride 0.9% w/v infusion fluid to give a volume of 50 mL. What is the concentration in mg/mL?

42. 100 mL of metronidazole suspension contains 4 g of the drug. How much do you give for a dose of 800 mg?

43. A patient weighing 80 kg is administered 100 mL of gentamycin 800 micrograms/mL over 30 minutes. What is the dose in mg/kg?

44. The treatment is pantoprazole 40 mg by intravenous infusion. Stock is a 40 mg vial of powder reconstituted with sodium chloride 0.9% w/v and diluted to 100 mL. What is the concentration of pantoprazole in the infusion fluid in microgram/mL?

45. The patient is prescribed a seven-day course of aciclovir 800 mg 5 times per day. How many grams of aciclovir in total will be consumed over the seven-day period?

46. 1.5 litres of saline is to be given over 10 hours using a 20 drop/mL giving set. What is the infusion rate in drops per minute?

47. A syringe driver contains 20 mg of morphine and 150 mg of promethazine in 6 mL of solution. The entire contents of the

syringe are infused in 24 hours. What is the dose rate for the promethazine in mg/hour?

48. The patient needs 28 units of insulin in the morning and 22 units in the evening, by subcutaneous injection. Stock is a 10 mL vial containing 100 units/mL. How many days supply of insulin are available per vial?

49. How much fluid will a 20 drop/mL giving set deliver over 12 hours if the infusion rate is set to 60 drops/minute?

50. Adrenaline is required. The stock is labelled as '1 in 10,000' (1 g in 10,000 mL) and you need to administer 1 mg. What volume do you give?

Nursing calculation mock test 2

Time allowed: one hour
NO CALCULATORS

1. The patient is written up for ibuprofen 1.2 g daily in four divided doses. How much ibuprofen is there in one dose?
2. The patient is started on quetiapine 25 mg b.d. on day 1, 50 mg b.d. on day 2, 100 mg b.d. on day 3 and 150 mg b.d. on day 4. How many milligrams of drug in total have been administered by the end of the fourth day?
3. Convert 0.0015 gram to milligrams.
4. Erythromycin is to be given 250 mg qid. What is the total daily dose?
5. The prescription asks for carvedilol 3.125 mg orally b.d. How many micrograms are there per dose?
6. Your patient is prescribed digoxin 500 microgram stat PO. The dose is repeated after 12 hours. How much digoxin has the patient received in total?
7. Phenobarbital elixir is to be given. The dose is 90 mg and the stock strength is 15 mg/5 mL. How much do you give?
8. An intravenous infusion of trimethoprim 200 mg is ordered. Stock is 20 mg/mL in 5 mL ampoules. How many ampoules are required?
9. A 10 mL syringe contains 20 mg of morphine. What is the concentration of morphine in mg/mL?
10. Dipyridamole oral suspension 50 mg/5 mL is prescribed. If the total daily dose is 300 mg, how many days' supply are there in a 150 mL bottle?
11. Convert 7.2 mg/day to micrograms per minute.
12. The prescription asks for betahistine 16 mg tds. Stock is 8 mg tablets. How many tablets does the patient take each day?
13. An infusion of dobutamine in 1.5 L of glucose 5% w/v commences at 0900 hours. If the infusion rate is 120 mL per hour at what time will the infusion finish?

14. An intravenous infusion of aciclovir is prescribed. A 500 mg vial of aciclovir powder is reconstituted with 20 mL of water. How much should be drawn up and added to the infusion bag for a dose of 400 mg?

15. If one litre of saline (0.9% w/v) is to be in infused over 12 hours using a standard giving set, how much should have been infused after 30 minutes, to the nearest millilitre?

16. 250 mL of Gelofusine is given IV stat over 15 minutes. What is the exact flow rate in mL/minute?

17. If an infusion pump delivers 120 mL in 90 minutes, what infusion rate is the pump set to in mL/hour?

18. A patient is to receive 500 mg of flucloxacillin. You have an oral solution of strength 125 mg/5 mL. What volume should you administer?

19. The prescription asks for 20 mg of oral morphine. Stock vials are 30 mg/5 mL. What volume is discarded after drawing up the drug? Give your answer to one decimal point.

20. Insulin syringes, with needles attached, come in sizes of 1 mL and are graduated in units (U) where 100 U = 1 mL. What is the volume of 35 units?

21. Bactroban ointment contains 2% w/w mupirocin as the active ingredient. How many milligrams of mupirocin are present in a 15 g tube of Bactroban?

22. Dextrose saline contains one-fifth as much sodium chloride as 0.9% w/v sodium chloride infusion fluid. What percentage is this?

23. How many grams of glucose will the patient receive if the order states 25 mL of 50% w/v glucose stat IV?

24. The prescription asks for gentamicin 5 mg/kg daily in divided doses every 8 hours. If the patient weighs 60 kg, how much should be administered in one dose?

25. One litre of sodium chloride 0.9% w/v is infused at a rate of 60 drops per minute using a 20 drop/mL giving set. How long should the infusion last in hours and minutes to the nearest minute?

26. Amiodarone 30 mg/mL is available in a 10 mL pre-filled syringe. How much amiodarone does it contain?

27. The prescription calls for dobutamine by intravenous infusion at 5 microgram/kg/minute. How many milligrams of dobutamine should have been infused after 10 hours if the patient weighs 72 kg?

28. Your patient has been prescribed quetiapine 450 mg in two divided doses. If the first dose is 250 mg, what is the second dose?

29. A 5 mg dose of salbutamol is given at a rate of 10 microgram/minute in 5% w/v glucose infusion fluid. How long with the infusion last to the nearest hour?

30. Quinine is given at a rate of 20 microgram/kg/minute. How much quinine is required per day for a patient weighing 50 kg?

31. The patient is written up for an intravenous infusion of mentronidazole 500 mg given over 20 minutes, every 8 hours. You have 5 mg/mL bags containing 100 mL metronidazole. How many bags do you need for the first day?

32. How much frusemide solution of strength 4 mg/mL should be administered for a 20 mg dose?

33. Amisulpride is prescribed. The stock strength is 100 mg/mL. How much is drawn up for a 500 mg dose?

34. The order is metronidazole 400 mg po tds for one week. How much metronidazole will be administered over this period?

35. Atenolol 150 microgram/kg is to be administered to a patient weighing 86 kg. Stock is 500 microgram/mL in10 mL ampoules. What volume do you draw up?

36. An injection of bupivacaine 0.25% w/v is to be administered. What is the concentration in mg/mL?

37. If 20 mg of diazepam is infused in 500 mL of sodium chloride 0.9% w/v infusion fluid, what is the concentration of the drug in microgram/mL?

38. 120 mg of morphine is to be given by continuous subcutaneous infusion every 24 hours. How much morphine should the patient have received after four hours?

39. The patient is written up for bumetanide by intravenous infusion. Two 500 microgram/mL 4 mL ampoules are drawn up and diluted with sodium chloride 0.9% w/v to give 500 mL of infusion fluid. What is the concentration of bumetanide in the infusion fluid in mg/L?

40. 1 gram of co-amoxiclav (Augmentin) is to be infused over 8 hours. You have 600 mg vials of powder for reconstitution. How many vials is this equivalent to (to two decimal places)?

41. 100 mL of reconstituted ciprofloxacin suspension contains 5 g of the drug. How much do you give for a dose of 500 mg?

42. 100 mL of metronidazole suspension contains 4 g of the drug. How much do you give for a dose of 500 mg?

43. If a 750 mg vial of cefuroxime powder is reconstituted water to give a solution of volume 7.5 mL, what is the concentration in mg/mL?

44. Citalopram oral drops are prescribed. A 15 mL bottle contains 600 mg of the drug. How many milligrams of the drug are present in one 0.05 mL drop?

45. 600 mL of fluid is to be infused over 4 hours using a 20 drops/mL giving set. Calculate the drops per minute.

46. An elixir of digoxin (Lanoxin-PG) contains 50 microgram per millilitre. How many 250 microgram doses are there in a 60 mL bottle of Lanoxin-PG?

47. A vial containing 500 mg of vancomycin powder is re-constituted with 'water for injection' to give 10 mL of solution. What dose is obtained by drawing up 2.5 mL of the vancomycin solution?

48. A syringe driver contains 40 mg of metoclopramide and 100 mg of morphine in 8 mL of solution. The entire contents of the syringe are infused in 24 hours. What is the dose rate for the morphine in mg/hour (to one decimal point)?

49. The patient self-administers 20 units of insulin by subcutaneous injection twice daily, using a reusable pen injector. How many days will two 3 mL 100 units/mL pen cartridges last?

50. You need to administer lignocaine at a rate of 1 mg/minute. You have a 500 mL bag of 5 % w/v glucose infusion fluid containing 1 gram of lignocaine. What is the infusion rate in mL/hour?

Nursing calculation mock test 3

Time allowed: one hour
NO CALCULATORS

1. The patient is prescribed 1 g amoxycillin per day in four divided doses. Stock is a 250 mg/5mL oral suspension. How many days supply are there in a 100 mL bottle?
2. Write 0.0625 milligram in micrograms.
3. The treatment is lithium carbonate 0.4–1.2 g daily in two divided doses. What is the maximum number of 200 mg tablets that can be given for one dose?
4. The controlled drugs cupboard contains two bottles of temazepam oral solution 10 mg/5 mL for a patient who takes 20 mg of the drug at bedtime. One bottle contains enough temazepam for 30 doses. What volume of temazepam would you expect to see recorded in the Ward Register on receipt of the medication (two full bottles)?
5. A child is to be given sodium valproate syrup 200 mg/5 mL. The dose is 20 mg/kg daily in two divided doses. Calculate the volume of one dose if the child weighs 16 kg.
6. Ciprofloxacin for infusion is available in 2 mg/mL glass vials. How much ciprofloxacin is there in a 200 mL vial?
7. You have a 3% w/v solution of a drug. The patient requires 60 mg. What volume do you give?
8. How many milligrams of phenytoin are there in a 15 mL dose of a 30 mg/5 mL suspension?
9. A patient requires an infusion of dopamine at a rate of 5 microgram/kg/minute for 12 hours. How many milligrams of dopamine are required if the patient weighs 92 kg?
10. Lignocaine 2% is to be injected. If the maximum dose is 200 mg what is the maximum volume?
11. A 300 mg bolus dose of amiodarone is given by intravenous injection over 4 minutes. Stock is a 30 mg/mL 10 mL pre-filled syringe. What is the flow rate in mL/minute?

12. An injection of 12 units of Mixtard insulin is ordered. Stock is 100 IU/mL 10 mL vial. You draw up 12 units into the insulin syringe. How many mL is this?

13. The patient is written up for an oral suspension of carbamazepine 20 mL tds. If the label on the bottle reads 'carbamazepine 100 mg/5 mL' what is the daily dose of carbamazepine in grams?

14. One gram of vancomycin is prescribed by intermittent intravenous infusion at a rate not to exceed 10 mg/minute. What is the minimum length of time for this infusion?

15. The patient is prescribed Jevity liquid to be PEG fed at a rate of 75 mL/hr for 20 hrs. How many 500 mL stock bottles will be required?

16. How many milligrams of lignocaine are there in 1 mL of 0.5% lignocaine?

17. Ranitidine in the form of sugar-free syrup has been prescribed for a child. The dose is 2 mg/kg, the stock strength is 75 mg/5 mL and the child weighs 22.5 kg. What volume should be drawn up?

18. How many micrograms of adrenaline are there in 1 mL of 1 in 10,000 adrenaline?

19. A 500 mg vial of vancomycin powder is reconstituted to a volume of 10 mL with sterile water for injection. What volume should be drawn up for a dose of 300 mg?

20. The patient is written up for a 15 mg/kg loading dose of phenytoin with a maintenance dose of 75 mg tds. The stock strength is 50 mg/mL. The patient weighs 60 kg. What volume of phenytoin is required for the first day of treatment?

21. Morphine is to be infused at a rate of 1.25 mg/hr. Stock is a 2 mg/mL 50 mL vial. What volume will be required for a 24-hour infusion?

22. How many grams of sodium chloride are there in a 500 mL bag of 0.9% w/v physiological saline?

23. How many grams of sodium chloride are there in a 1 L bag of 0.18% w/v sodium chloride and 4% glucose solution?

24. If 1 L of 0.9% physiological saline contains 150 mmol (millimoles) of sodium chloride, how many mmol are there in 1L of 0.18% sodium chloride solution?

25. An injection of enoxaparin 1.5 mg/kg is to be given. The patient weighs 60 kg. Stock is a 1 mL pre-filled enoxaparin 100 mg/mL syringe with graduation marks every 2.5 mg. How many graduations will have to be expelled before you can give the injection?

26. A patient-controlled analgesia (PCA) infusion pump contains morphine 1 mg/mL. The patient receives a bolus dose of 1 mL when the button is pressed. If the minimum period between doses ('lock-out time') is set to 6 minutes, what is the maximum dose of morphine available to the patient in mg/hr?

27. The PCA prescription is for fentanyl 25 microgram/mL with a 20 microgram/6 minute lock-out time. What is the volume of each bolus dose?

28. An injection of 10,000 units of heparin is ordered. Stock is a 25,000 units/mL in a 1 mL ampoule. What volume should be drawn up?

29. The patient is to receive an infusion of heparin 1,000 units/mL. You draw up two 5 mL ampoules, four 1 mL ampoules and a further 0.4 mL from a 1 mL ampoule. The heparin is diluted to 24 mL with 0.9% saline and given at a rate of 2 mL/hr via a syringe driver. Calculate the dose rate in units/hour.

30. The patient is prescribed an infusion of heparin at 1,000 units/hr. In stock is a 5 mL 5000 units/mL ampoule which is diluted to 50 mL with 0.9% saline. What is the rate of the infusion in mL/hr?

31. The treatment is an intravenous infusion of imipenem with cilastatin. The total daily dose should not exceed 50 mg/kg/day or 4 g/day. What is the total daily dose for a patient weighing 82 kg?

32. How many milligrams of potassium chloride are there in 1 mL of 15% potassium chloride solution?

33. What is the difference in milligrams per day between 5 mg

tds and 5 mg total daily dose?
34. How many grams of paracetamol are there in 10 mL of paediatric oral suspension of strength120 mg/5 mL?
35. The treatment is 3.054 g lithium citrate oral solution daily in two divided doses. Stock is an oral solution containing 509 mg/5 mL. What volume do you measure out for one dose?
36. A patient is to receive an intravenous infusion of aminophylline at a rate of 36 mg/hour. Stock is a 25 mg/mL 10 mL ampoule of aminophylline mixed with glucose 5% w/v to give 500 mL of intravenous infusion fluid. What is the infusion rate in mL/hour?
37. A one litre bottle of Jevity liquid is fed via a pump. The rate is set to 100 mL/hr and the pump is switched on at 2200 hours. The rate is increased at 0200 hours. If the feed finished at 0700 hours what was the rate increased to?
38. A child is to receive an infusion of insulin at a rate of 0.1 units/kg/hour. The syringe pump contains 50 units of insulin in 50 mL of 0.9 % sodium chloride. At what speed in mL/hour should the pump be set at for a child weighing 40 kg?
39. Convert 1 microgram/minute to mg/day.
40. 500 mL of sodium chloride 0.9% w/v is to be given subcutaneously over 10 hours using a 20 drop/mL giving set. What is the infusion rate in drops per minute to the nearest drop?
41. What is a 0.05% w/v solution in micrograms/mL?
42. The prescription is for a sugar-free oral solution of frusemide. What is the concentration of the stock in mg/mL if a 5 mL dose contains 40 mg of the drug?
43. The daily therapeutic dose of ceftriaxone for infants and children up to 12 years is 20–50 mg/kg body weight. What is the maximum daily dose for a 10-year-old child weighing 38 kg?
44. The weight of a child up to age 10 years can be estimated from the equation: Weight in kg = 2 × (age + 4). Estimate the weight of a seven-year-old child.
45. The treatment is 20 mg of omeprazole daily PO for 8 weeks.

How many grams of omeprazole will be consumed in total?

46. A 1 g vial of cefotaxime powder is reconstituted with 4.2 mL of water for injection. If the volume of the solution is 5 mL how much water has the powder displaced?

47. A 250 mg vial of flucloxacillin powder is reconstituted with 9.7 mL of water for injection. The displacement volume is 0.3 mL. What volume do you draw up for a dose of 250 mg?

48. A 500 mg vial of vancomycin powder is reconstituted with 9.5 mL of water for injection. The displacement volume is 0.5 mL. What volume do you draw up for a dose of 300 mg?

49. A 750 mg vial of cefuroxime powder is reconstituted with 5.5 mL of water for injection. If the displacement volume is 0.5 mL what volume do you draw up for a dose of 600 mg?

50. A patient weighing 80 kg is written up for a continuous intravenous infusion of dopamine at a rate of 10 microgram/kg/minute. Two 10 mL 40 mg/mL vials of dopamine are diluted to 500 mL with 0.9% sodium chloride. What rate should the infusion pump be set to in mL/hr?

Answers to tests

Basic maths self-assessment test

Remedial level

1. Twenty-five
2. Four thousand and sixty
3. Nine hundred and eighty thousand one hundred and seven
4. 3030
5. 1,210,000
6. 12,500
7. 0.3
8. two hundreds; 200
9. 75 cents
10. 11.30 pm

Level 1

11. 20
12. 1020
13. 136
14. 288
15. 63
16. 15
17. $3.77
18. 5 degrees
19. 23,400
20. $11,250

Level 2

21.	$7^{3}/_{4}$	26.	$1020
22.	3	27.	$^{1}/_{5}$
23.	15.65	28.	0.45
24.	27	29.	250 mg
25.	76	30.	1.46

Answers to Chapter 1 test exercises

Test 1

1.	1168	5.	433
2.	9042	6.	18,050
3.	2009	7.	1127
4.	27,550	8.	1112

Test 2

1.	63	6.	95
2.	96	7.	99
3.	120	8.	300
4.	92	9.	1000
5.	450	10.	132

Test 3

1.	806	6.	10,000
2.	2528	7.	5511
3.	1200	8.	5082
4.	5080	9.	39,975
5.	425	10.	702

Test 4

1.	4	5.	410
2.	62	6.	59
3.	113	7.	244
4.	53	8.	125

Test 5

1.	30	6.	6
2.	31	7.	38
3.	44	8.	67
4.	45	9.	61
5.	20	10.	206

Test 6

1.	14	7.	9
2.	13	8.	56
3.	10	9.	10
4.	2	10.	6
5.	14	11.	6
6.	9	12.	14

Test 7

1.	24	7.	39
2.	2	8.	57
3.	5	9.	3
4.	44	10.	36
5.	10	11.	5
6.	21	12.	9000

Test 8

1. 1 2 3 6
2. 1 2 5 10
3. 1 2 3 4 8 16 32
4. 1 2 3 5 6 9 10 15 18 30 45 90
5. 1 2 4 5 10 20 25 50 100 125 250 500
6. 8
7. 15
8. 4
9. 50
10. 25

Test 9

1. 2×3
2. 2×3×5
3. 3×3×7
4. 2×2×3×5×7

5. 3×3×3×3
6. 2×2×2×3×3×3
7. 5×5×5
8. 7×7×7

Test 10

1. 2 4 6 8
2. 12 24 36 48
3. 20 40 60 80
4. 25 50 75 100
5. 100 200 300 400

6. 6
7. 60
8. 72
9. 150
10. 200

Answers to Chapter 1 questions

1. 2022
2. 610
3. 195
4. 2592
5. 108
6. 64
7. 5625
8. 148 473
9. 11
10. 39
11. 224
12. 72
13. 130
14. 20
15. 100

16. 16
17. 54
18. 80
19. 26
20. 150
21. 1 2 4 5 10 20
22. 2 and 5
23. 1 2 3 6 7 14 21 42
24. 2, 3 and 7
25. 6 12 18 24 30 36
26. 9 18 27 36 45 54
27. 18
28. 100
29. 250
30. 60

Answers to Chapter 2 test exercises

Test 11

1. $\frac{1}{2}$
2. $\frac{3}{4}$
3. $\frac{1}{3}$
4. $\frac{5}{9}$
5. $\frac{2}{3}$

6. $\frac{3}{5}$
7. $\frac{1}{10}$
8. $\frac{19}{20}$
9. $\frac{2}{3}$
10. $\frac{2}{5}$

Test 12

1. $\frac{7}{8}$
2. $\frac{5}{6}$
3. $\frac{3}{10}$
4. $\frac{7}{12}$

5. 1
6. $\frac{1}{2}$
7. $\frac{2}{3}$
8. $\frac{2}{5}$

Test 13

1. 15
2. 12
3. 16

4. $\frac{7}{15}$
5. $\frac{11}{12}$
6. $\frac{7}{16}$

Test 14

1. $\frac{3}{4}$
2. $\frac{2}{3}$
3. $\frac{2}{5}$

4. $\frac{7}{8}$
5. $\frac{16}{50}$
6. $\frac{7}{100}$

Test 15

1. $\frac{2}{27}$
2. $\frac{8}{45}$
3. $\frac{16}{63}$
4. $\frac{2}{27}$
5. $\frac{3}{500}$

6. $\frac{1}{2}$
7. $\frac{1}{3}$
8. $\frac{1}{4}$
9. $\frac{2}{27}$
10. $\frac{3}{10}$

Test 16

1. $^2/_3$
2. $^3/_5$
3. $^3/_4$
4. $^1/_2$
5. $^5/_6$

6. $^2/_5$
7. $^1/_{25}$
8. $^1/_{200}$
9. $^3/_{20}$
10. $^2/_3$

Test 17

1. $^{25}/_{12}$
2. $^1/_6$
3. $^{15}/_8$
4. $^1/_2$

5. $^{49}/_{10}$
6. $^8/_3$
7. $^{20}/_9$
8. 50

Test 18

1. $^7/_4$
2. $^{11}/_2$
3. $^{17}/_6$
4. $^{27}/_8$
5. $^{67}/_{10}$

6. $^{119}/_{100}$
7. $^6/_5$
8. $^{12}/_5$
9. $^7/_5$

Test 19

1. $4^1/_2$
2. $5^3/_4$
3. $5^1/_3$

4. $16^2/_3$
5. $5^1/_4$
6. $12^1/_2$

Test 20

1. $2^1/_2$
2. $4^1/_2$
3. $3^1/_2$
4. $10^4/_5$

5. $7^1/_2$
6. $^3/_{20}$
7. $^1/_{36}$
8. $^1/_{24}$

Test 21

1.	$1^2/_5$	9.	$^9/_{20}$
2.	$4^1/_4$	10.	$^1/_2$
3.	8	11.	$^1/_4$
4.	30	12.	$^1/_{12}$
5.	64	13.	$^1/_5$
6.	72	14.	$3^3/_5$
7.	$^5/_8$	15.	$^1/_{400}$
8.	$^1/_4$		

Test 22

1.	3	6.	5
2.	14	7.	3
3.	8	8.	1
4.	8	9.	5
5.	8		

Test 23

1.	22.5	6.	a, c, b, d
2.	0.275	7.	a, d, c, b
3.	0.02	8.	b, c, a, d
4.	200.075	9.	a, c, b, d
5.	d, b, c, a		

Test 24

1.	1589.7	5.	17 170.3
2.	769.2105	6.	25
3.	3172.9	7.	5.8
4.	0.0175	8.	100

Test 25

1.	8.96	6.	160
2.	20.02	7.	3

3. 0.3553
4. 0.005 44
5. 1.5015

8. 100.2
9. 2032
10. 14,000

Test 26

1. 1.7
2. 12.45
3. 8.031 25
4. 170
5. 33.3
6. 11.1

7. 6
8. 60
9. 1.2
10. 62,500
11. 20,000
12. 0.016

Test 27

1. 6.08
2. 0.38543

3. 0.8
4. 7.96

Test 28

1. 4.17
2. 14.2857
3. 10.4
4. 44
5. 81

6. 160
7. 66
8. 17
9. 3
10. 133

Test 29

1. $^3/_5$
2. $^3/_4$
3. $^5/_8$
4. $^9/_{10}$
5. $^1/_{1000}$

6. $^2/_{25}$
7. $^{19}/_{20}$
8. $1^3/_4$
9. $2^3/_8$

Test 30

1. 0.3
2. 0.25

6. 0.875
7. 0.85

3. 0.4
4. 1.25
5. 0.12

8. 0.105
9. 0.18

Test 31

1. $^1/_5$ and 0.2
2. $^1/_4$ and 0.25
3. $^1/_{10}$ and 0.1
4. $^3/_4$ and 0.75
5. $^9/_{10}$ and 0.9

6. $^9/_{20}$ and 0.45
7. $^7/_{20}$ and 0.35
8. $^{11}/_{50}$ and 0.22
9. $^1/_{50}$ and 0.02

Test 32

1. 90
2. 60
3. 125

4. 25
5. 10%
6. 9000

Test 33

1. 50%
2. 75%
3. 100%
4. 20%
5. 12.5%

6. 1.5%
7. 105%
8. 0.5%
9. 36%
10. 85%

Answers to Chapter 2 questions

1. $^3/_5$
2. $^2/_9$
3. $^3/_8$
4. $^2/_7$
5. $^1/_{32}$
6. $^7/_{20}$
7. $3^6/_7$
8. $^9/_2$
9. $6^1/_8$
10. $^1/_{20}$

11. 0.625, $^3/_4$, 0.905, 0.95, 1.2
12. 2.2
13. 5
14. 0.72
15. 0.0625
16. 5000
17. 8.38
18. 0.167
19. $^1/_{16}$
20. 12.5

Answers to Chapter 3 test exercises

Test 34

1. 25 micrograms
2. 1 g
3. 330 micrograms

4. 1.275 g
5. 0.42 mg

Test 35

1. 1 g
2. 2.5 g
3. 1.25 g
4. 4.5 mg
5. 500 mg
6. 250 mg

7. 325 micrograms
8. 10 mg
9. 1.2 kg
10. 50 mg
11. 500 micrograms
12. 12 micrograms

Test 36

1. 500 mL
2. 50 mL
3. 1250 mL
4. 125 mL
5. 2 L

6. 4.05 L
7. 0.005 L
8. 0.25 L
9. 0.0105 L
10. 10 mL

Test 37

1. kg
2. L
3. mg
4. mcg or μg
5. kg

6. g
7. mcg
8. g
9. L

Test 38

1. 2.1 g
2. 1.65 g

5. 0.9 mg
6. 435 mg

3. 3 g
4. 0.7 g

7. 0.6005 g
8. 675 micrograms

Test 39

1. 1 g
2. 1.5 g
3. 12.5 mg
4. 2 mg
5. 0.3 kg

6. 5 mg
7. 200 micrograms
8. 7.5 micrograms
9. 0.5 micrograms
10. 2.5 g

Test 40

1. 0625 hrs
2. 1705 hrs
3. 9.50 pm
4. 10.10 am
5. 7.30 pm
6. 0145 hrs

7. 1 hr 33 min
8. 18 mins
9. 132 secs
10. ²/₃
11. 54 secs
12. 20 secs

Test 41

1. 5.5 mL
2. 1.5 mL
3. 1.2 mL

4. 2.5 mL
5. 0.55 mL
6. 2.8 mL

Test 42

1. 0.6 mL
2. 1.5 mL
3. 0.7 mL

4. 0.65 mL
5. 1.4 mL
6. 0.95 mL

Answers to Chapter 3 questions

1. 2 g
2. 400 mg
3. 250 micrograms

11. 150 mg
12. 1.1 L
13. 1.025 L

4.	10 micrograms	14.	62 mL
5.	80 mg	15.	577.5 mL
6.	7.5 mL	16.	23:30 hrs
7.	5.5 g	17.	08:30 hrs
8.	0.95 mL	18.	13:15 hrs
9.	7.65432 g	19.	0.05 mL
10.	20 mg	20.	4 mL

Answers to Chapter 4 test exercises

Test 43

1.	3 tablets	6.	3 tablets
2.	2 tablets	7.	4 tablets
3.	15 mL	8.	10 mL
4.	10 mL	9.	400 mg
5.	4 mL	10.	1.25 mg

Test 44

1.	a) 0.5 mL	3.	a) 5 mL
	b) 0.75 mL		b) 2 mL
	c) 1 mL		c) 2.5 mL
	d) 1.5 mL		d) 1 mL
2.	a) 3 mL	4.	a) 20 mL
	b) 2 mL		b) 15 mL
	c) 1 mL		c) 1 mL
	d) 0.4 mL		d) 5 mL

Test 45

1.	a) 100	2.	a) 67 dpm
	b) 80		b) 83 dpm
	c) 16		c) 28 dpm
	d) 30		d) 42 dpm

Test 46

1.	10 mg/mL	7.	20 g
2.	20 mg/mL	8.	1.875 g
3.	2 mg/mL	9.	750 units
4.	40 mg/mL	10.	a) 50 mg/mL
5.	50 mg/mL		b) 2 mg/mL
6.	25 g		

Test 47 with explanations

1. a) 1.6 mg/mL
    b) 267 mcg/min
    c) 0.267 mg/mL
    d) 16.0 mg/hr
    e) 10 mL/hr
    a) 400 mg in 250 mL = $^{400}/_{250}$ = $^{40}/_{25}$ = $^{8}/_{5}$ = $1^{3}/_{8}$ = 1.6 mg/mL
    b) Rate = 3 mcg/kg/min × 89 kg = 267 mcg/min
    c) 267 mcg/min = 0.267 mg/min
    d) 0.267 mg/min × 60 min = 2.67 × 6 = 16.02 = 16.0 mg/hr to one decimal place
    e) 16 mg/hr ÷ 1.6 mg/mL in a) = 160 ÷ 16 = 10 mL/hr
    If you find e) difficult, take a one-hour period, then e) becomes 16 mg ÷ 1.6 mg/mL in 1 hour; 1.6 mg/mL means 1.6 mg in 1 mL or 16 mg in 10 mL; 10 mL in one hour = 10 mL/hr

2. a) 75 mg
    b) 3000 mcg/hr
    c) 3 mg/hr
    d) 0.15 mg/mL
    e) 20 mL/hr
    f) 25 hours
    a) One 3 mL ampoule = 3 mL × 25 mg/mL = 75 mg
    b) Rate = 40 mcg/kg/min × 75 kg = 3000 mcg/min
    c) 3000 mcg/hr = 3 mg/hr
    d) 75 mg/500 mL = $^{75}/_{500}$ = $^{15}/_{100}$ = 0.15 mg/mL
    e) 3 mg/hr ÷ 0.15 mg/mL = 300 ÷ 15 = 20 mL/hr
    f) 500 mL at 20 mL/hr = $^{500}/_{20}$ = 25 hours

3. 200 drops/min

Volume = $\dfrac{100 \text{ mL} \times \text{drip factor (60)}}{\text{Time} = 30 \text{ minutes}}$

= 200 d.p.m.

4. 120 mL/hr

Stock is 0.2% w/v = 0.2 g/100 mL = 200 mg/100 mL = 2 mg/mL

Rate = 4 mg/min ÷ 2 mg/mL = 2 mL/min or 120 mL/hr

5. a) 500 mg

b) 10 mL

c) 4 amps

d) 260 mL

e) 130 mL/hr

a) 5 mg/kg × 100 kg = 500 mg

b) Dose prescribed = 500 mg; dose per measure = 50 mg
$^{500}/_{50} \times 1$ mL = 10 mL

c) 10 mL ÷ 3 mL/ampoule = $3^{1}/_{3}$ ampoules; round up to 4 amp

d) Total volume = 250 mL diluent + 10 mL drug = 260 mL

e) Rate in mL/hr − 260 mL/2 hr = 130 mL/hr

6. a) 27 mg

b) 2.7 mL

a) 1.5 mcg/kg × 100 kg × 60 min/hr × 3 hr = 150 × 180 = 27000 mcg = 27 mg

b) Stock is a 10 mg/mL. Dose prescribed = 27 mg; dose per measure = 10 mg. $^{27}/_{10} \times 1$ mL = 2.7 mL

7. a) 4.25 g

b) 2.125 vials

c) 521.25 mL

d) 2.2 mL/min

a) Dose prescribed = 50 mg/kg × 85 kg = 4250 mg = 4.25 g

b) Each ampoule contains 200 mg/mL × 10 mL = 2000 mg = 2g. Exact number of vials required = 4.25 ÷ 2 = 2.125 vials

c) Volume = 500 mL + 2.125 vials × 10 mL/vial = 521.25 mL

d) Infusion time = 4 hr × 60 min/hr = 240 mins; infusion rate 521.25 mL ÷ 240 mins = 2.2 mL/min to one decimal point

8. 100 hrs
   5 mcg/kg/min = 5 × 83 × 60 = 24900 mcg/hr = 24.9 mg/hr.
   Stock = 20 mL × 125 mg/mL = 2500 mg; at 24.9 mg/hr = 100 hrs

Test 48

1. 2230 hours
2. 250 mL/hr

Test 49

1. mcg/kg/min
   a) 1
   b) 0.5
   c) 2.5
   d) 12.5

Answers to Chapter 4 questions

1. 4 tablets
2. 2 mL
3. 3 vials
4. 10 mL
5. 15 mL
6. 1 mL
7. 18 mL
8. 37.5 mL
9. 4 minutes
10. 80 mL/hr
11. 2.5 mg/hr
12. 370 mg/hr
13. 8.2 mL
14. 25 mL/hr
15. 0.1 g (100 mg)
16. 56 drops/min
17. 50 mg/mL
18. 10 mg/mL
19. 250 mL
20. 3 mg/mL

Test 50

1. 4 tablets
2. 400 mg
3. 7.5 g
4. 4 g
5. none
6. 12 days
7. 3 g
8. 20 mg
9. 4 packs
10. 40 tablets
11. 30 mg

Test 51

1.	B	11.	A
2.	A	12.	A
3.	C	13.	C
4.	A	14.	C
5.	B	15.	C
6.	C	16.	B
7.	A	17.	A
8.	A	18.	A
9.	C	19.	B
10.	B	20.	C

Test 52

1. Ciprofloxacin = Ciproxin. 400 mg/200 mL; so *200 mL/hr*
2. Baclofen = Lioresal 5 mg/5 mL. 3 doses of 10 mg = 2 *spoonfuls/dose*
3. Enoxaparin = Clexane; dose 0.5 mg/kg = 0.5 × 60 = 30 mg; stock 40 mg/0.4 mL = 10 mg/0.1 mL; *expel 0.1 mL*
4. Impenem with cilstatin = Primaxin IV; dose 1.5 mg/day = 3 *vials per day*
5. Maxolon = metoclopramide; 20 mg; bolus dose = (20 ÷ 10) × 2 mL = *4 mL*
6. 20 mg Prozac = 5 mL of fluoxetine
7. Carbamazepine = Tegretol; Four 5 mL spoonfuls = 4 × 100 mg = 400 mg
8. GTN – glyceryl trinitrate = Nitrolingual pump spray for as required use

Test 53

1. False. The patient's given names are Christopher and John and his family name is Jones. Be on the alert for similar names.
2. True. He is prescribed 1 gm paracetamol four times a day.
3. True. He has had the dose for 5 July.
4. False. The medication has aleady been given. It is next due at mid-day.
5. False. Perindopril is to be administered 1 hour before breakfast.

Test 54

1. True. Correct patient but check other details when the patient's name is a common one.
2. False. The dose is 25 *micrograms*, not milligrams. It is safer to write mcg in full.
3. True. 75 mg diclofenac is given twice a day.
4. False. The next dose is due in the evening.
5. False. Gliclazide 30 mg is a sustained released tablet and must not be crushed.

Test 55

1. False. The patient's name is Xiang Le. Always confirm the name if you are not familiar with it.
2. False. Breaking a tablet might not provide an accurate dose. Give two 62.5 microgram tablets.
3. True. The next dose will depend on the level of the drug in her blood.
4. True. Administer a 1 mg tablet and a 3 mg tablet, or two 2 mg tablets.
5. False. Do not crush sustained release tablets.

Test 56

1. False. The dose is 30 mg not mcg.

2. True. This is the corrrect dose.
3. True. It is permissable to split a scored tablet, but make sure that it splits equally.
4. False. Even if medications appear to be the same and belong to the same drug grouping, they might not be interchangeable. Do not substitute without an order.
5. False. Budesonide is administered by inhalation.

Test 57

1. True. But observe the specific requirements for this medication: it is administered 30 minutes before breakfast and Mrs Luciano is to remain upright for at least 30 minutes.
2. False. The next dose is due seven days later on 19 October.
3. False. Never substitute one drug for another because the names sound similar, even if they belong to the same drug grouping.
4. False. For brevity it is acceptable to write the trade name of compound medications.

Answers to the nursing numerical test

See also the expanded answers below.

1.	C	16.	B
2.	B	17.	A
3.	C	18.	B
4.	D	19.	A
5.	D	20.	C
6.	A	21.	B
7.	C	22.	C
8.	B	23.	D
9.	B	24.	A
10.	D	25.	B
11.	C	26.	B

12. A	27. D
13. A	28. C
14. D	29. D
15. A	30. A

Expanded answers for the nursing numerical test

1. 1630 hrs − 0700 hrs = 0930 = 9.5 hrs (C).
2. 400 mg ÷ 1000 mg/g = 0.4 g (B).
3. $^{32}/_{40} \times 100 \% = \ ^{32}/_{4} \times 10 = 8 \times 10 = 80\%$ (C).
4. 2200 mL ÷ 1000 mL/L = 2.2 L (D).
5. $^{15}/_{9} = \ ^{5}/_{3} = 1^{2}/_{3} = 1.6666 = 1.667$ to three decimal points (D).
6. 25.4 ÷ 0.04 = 2540 ÷ 4 = 635 (A).
7. 0.05 mg × 1000 mcg/mg = 50 micrograms (C).
8. 1 drop every 3 seconds and 60 seconds in every minute = 60 ÷ 3 drops per minute = 20 dpm. Each drop = 0.1 mL = 20 × 0.1 mL/min = 2 mL/min = 2 × 60 mL/hr = 120 mL/hr (B).
9. 1 gram = 1000 milligrams. 200 mg as a fraction of 1 g is $^{200}/_{1000} = \ ^{2}/_{10} = \ ^{1}/_{5}$ (B).
10. In cents: 450 c − 85 c = 365 c = \$3.65 (D).
11. Convert 10 g to kg then add it to 1 kg: 10 g = $^{10}/_{1000}$ kg = 0.01 kg; 1 kg + 0.01 kg = 1.01 kg (C).
12. 500 × $^{3}/_{4}$ = 125 × 3 = 375 mL (A).
13. Total students = 42 + 8 = 50. 8 men: $^{8}/_{50} \times 100\% = 8 \times 2 = 16\%$ men (A).
14. 25 ÷ $^{5}/_{6}$ = 25 × $^{6}/_{5}$ = 5 × 6 = 30 (D).
15. 5 ÷ 8 = 0. 6 2 5   (A)
    8⌐5.^{5}0^{2}0^{4}0
16. Work out the brackets first: 4(4 × 3 − 2) = 4(12 − 2) = 4(10) = 4 × 10 = 40 (B).
17. 3 $^{3}/_{16}$ × 1$^{1}/_{3}$ = $^{48+3}/_{16}$ × $^{4}/_{3}$ = $^{51}/_{16}$ × $^{4}/_{3}$ = $^{17}/_{4}$ = 4$^{1}/_{4}$ = 4.25 (A).
18. 60% as a fraction = $^{60}/_{100}$ = $^{6}/_{10}$ = $^{3}/_{5}$ (B).
19. 1700 hrs − 0730 hrs = 0930 hrs; less 30 min = 9 hrs (A).
20. 20 ÷ 0.004 = 20000 ÷ 4 = 5000 (C).
21. 22% as a decimal = 22 ÷ 100 = 0.22 (B).

22. 1.8 g ÷ 4 = 0.45 g × 1000 mg/g = 450 mg (C).
23. 7 = 5 + 1 +1 = 7 mg in 3 tablets (D).
24. Every 6 hours = 4 doses per day. 500 mg × 4 doses/day = 2000 mg/day = 2g (A).
25. One litre = 1000 mL to be given at a rate of 125 mL/hr. 1000 mL ÷ 125 mL/hr = $^{1000}/_{125}$ hr = 8 hr (B).
26. 30 mg ÷ 12 = $^{30}/_{12}$ = $^{15}/_{6}$ = $^{5}/_{2}$ = 2.5 mg (B).
27. 90 kg × 10% = 90 × $^{10}/_{100}$ = 9 kg; 90 − 9 = 81 kg (D).
28. $^{5}/_{6}$ = $^{10}/_{12}$ = $^{10}/_{24}$ so not D nor A, which leaves B or C. B = $^{14}/_{18}$ = $^{7}/_{9}$ so not B. C = $^{25}/_{30}$ = $^{5}/_{6}$ (C).
29. 4% of 2 L = $^{4}/_{100}$ × 2000 mL = 4 × 20 = 80 mL (D).
30. 1 g − 25 mg = 1000 − 25 = 975 mg = 0.975 g (A).

Answers to mock test 1

See also the expanded answers which follow.

1.	300 mg	26.	75 mL/hr
2.	25 microgram	27.	180 mg
3.	6 capsules	28.	20 mL
4.	30 g	29.	5000 units
5.	Half a tablet	30.	7.2 mL
6.	1.2 g	31.	0.375 mg
7.	16 mg	32.	16.7 mL
8.	15 mL	33.	80 mg
9.	8 mg/mL	34.	Two tablets
10.	1 g	35.	125 mL/hr
11.	12 mg/hr	36.	7.2 mg
12.	3.5 g	37.	25 mg/min
13.	8 tablets/day	38.	1.44 L/day
14.	5 hours	39.	120 mL/hr
15.	4 mL	40.	1 L approx
16.	125 mL	41.	10 mg/mL
17.	10 mL	42.	20 mL
18.	10 mg	43.	1 mg/kg
19.	1.6 mL	44.	400 micrograms/mL

20. 0.38 mL	45. 28 g
21. 600 micrograms	46. 50 drops/min
22. 0.1 micrograms	47. 6.25 mg/hr
23. 2.8 g	48. 20 days
24. 10 g	49. 2.16 L
25. 37.5 mg	50. 10 mL

Mock test 1 expanded answers

1. 700 mg − 200 mg − 200 mg = *300 mg.*
2. 0.025 mg × 1000 mcg/mg = *25 micrograms.*
3. 1.2 mg = 1.2 mg × 1000 mcg/mg =1200 micrograms. 1200 ÷ 200 = *6 capsules.*
4. First 10 days: 500 mg × 10 = 5 g.
   Second 10 days: (500 + 500) mg × 10 = 10 g.
   Third 10 days: (500 + 500 + 500) mg × 10 = 15 g.
   Total = 30 g.
5. $^{40}/_{80}$ = *half a tablet.*
6. 600 mg × 2 = 1200 mg = *1.2 g.*
7. 2 mg/dose × 4 doses/day × 2 days = *16 mg.*
8. Dose prescribed = 150 mg; dose per measure = 50 mg.
   $^{150}/_{50}$ × 5 mL = 3 × 5 mL = *15 mL.*
9. $^{40mg}/_{5ml}$ = *8 mg/mL.*
10. 5% w/v = 5 g/100 mL = 1g /20 mL. So 20 mL contains *1 g.*
11. 200 micrograms/minute = 0.2 mg/minute. 0.2 mg/min × 60 min/hr = *12 mg/hr.*
12. 250 mg b.d. = 250 mg twice daily = 500 mg/day. Converting to grams: 0.5 g/day for 7 days = *3.5 g.*
13. 2 tablets q.d.s. = 2 tablets 4 times daily = *8 tablets/day.*
14. $^{500ml}/_{100ml/hr}$ = *5 hours.*
15. Dose prescribed = 160 mg; dose per measure = 40 mg.
    $^{160}/_{40}$ × 1 mL = *4 mL* (note: the measure is 1 mL not 6 mL).
16. 2.5 hours × 50 mL/hr = *125 mL.*
17. Dose prescribed = 10 mg; dose per measure = 5 mg. $^{10}/_{5}$ × 5 mL = 10 mL.

18. 100 mg/5ml = 20 mg/mL; volume administered = 0.5 mL.
    0.5 mL × 20 mg/mL = *10 mg*.
19. Dose prescribed = 80 mg; dose per measure = 50 mg. $^{80}/_{50}$ × 1
    = *1.6 mL* (note: the measure is 1 mL not 2 mL).
20. Dose prescribed = 150 mcg; dose per measure = 400 mg/mL.
    $^{150}/_{400}$ × 1 = $^{15}/_{40}$ = $^{3}/_{8}$ = 0.375 mL = *0.38 mL* (to the nearest
    100th of a mL = to two decimal places.)
21. 0.6 mg × 1000 mcg/mg = *600 micrograms*.
22. 20 drops per mL; 2 microgram per mL. 20 drops = 2 mcg so
    1 drop = *0.1 microgram*.
23. 70% w/w means 70 g/100 g: 4 g × $^{70}/_{100}$ = $^{280}/_{100}$ = *2.8 g*.
24. 20% w/v means 20 g/100 mL: 50 g × $^{20}/_{100}$ = $^{1000}/_{100}$ = *10 g*.
25. 500 micrograms × 75 = 0.5 mg × 75 = *37.5 mg*.
26. $^{48}/_{80}$ × 1 litre cancels to $^{6}/_{10}$ × 1 L = 0.6 L. 0.6 L per 8 hours
    = 600 mL/8 hr = *75 mL/hr*.
27. 0.5 mg/min × 60 min/hr × 6 hr = 5 × 6 × 6 mg = *180 mg*.
28. 600 mg ÷ 3 doses = 200 mg; $^{200}/_{50}$ × 5 mL = *20 mL*.
29. 25 000 units in 1.0 mL and we have 0.2 mL. $^{0.2}/_{1.0}$ × 25 000 =
    $^{2}/_{10}$ × 25 000 = 2 × 2500 = *5000 units*.
30. 100 mcg/kg/hr × 60 kg × 12 mcg = 1000 × 6 × 12 mcg =
    72 mg. Stock: 10 mg/mL; 72 mg ÷ 10 mg/mL = *7.2 mL*.
31. 1.5 mg ÷ 4 = 0.375 mg.
    ```
       0. 3 7 5
    4|1.¹5³0²0
    ```
32. Dose prescribed = 1 g; dose per measure = 1.2 g. $^{1}/_{1.2}$ × 20 mL
    = $^{20}/_{1.2}$ = $^{200}/_{12}$ = $^{100}/_{6}$ = $^{50}/_{3}$ = $16^{2}/_{3}$ = 16.667 = *16.7 mL* to one
    decimal place.
33. 200 doses × 400 microgram/dose = 200 × $^{400}/_{1000}$ mg =
    200 × $^{4}/_{10}$ mg = 20 × 4 mg = *80 mg*.
34. 5 mg/kg × 80 kg = 400 mg. Stock is 200 mg tablets = 2.
35. We have 5 mL × 96 mg/mL = 480 mg in 125 mL of fluid.
    Dose = 8 mg/min = $^{8}/_{480}$ × 125 mL/min = $^{1}/_{60}$ × 125 =
    $^{125}/_{60}$ mL/min = *125 mL/hr*.
36. 100 micrograms × 24 × 3 = 100 × 72 = 7200 microgram =
    7.2 mg.

37. 1 g per 40 minutes = 1000 mg/40 min = $^{1000}/_{40}$ = $^{100}/_{4}$ = *25 mg/min.*
38. 1 mL/min = 1 × 60 × 24 mL/day = 1440 mL/day = *1.44 L/day.*
39. 0.2% = 0.2 g/100 mL = 200 mg/100 mL = 2 mg/mL.
    Rewrite this as 4 mg/2 mL. Rate = 4 mg/min = 2 mL/min = *120 mL/hr.*
40. 14 drops in 30 seconds = 28 drops/minute. We have 20 drops per mL giving set = $^{28\ drops/min}/_{20\ drop/mL}$ = $^{14}/_{10}$ mL/min = 1.4 mL/min.
    (Check: 1.4 × 20 = 28.) Multiply by 60 minutes to give mL/hour: 1.4 mL/min × 60 min/hr = 14 × 6 mL/hr = 84 mL/hr. 84 mL/hr × 12 hr = 1008 mL = *1 L approx.*
41. 500 mg/50 mL = *10 mg/mL.*
42. $^{800}/_{4000}$ × 100 mL = $^{8}/_{40}$ × 100 = $^{8}/_{4}$ × 10 mL = *20 mL.*
    Check: 800 mg is one-fifth of 4 g. One-fifth of 100 mL = 20 mL.
43. 800 micrograms × 100 = 80 000 micrograms = 80 mg. 80 mg ÷ 80 kg = *1 mg/kg.*
44. $^{40}/_{100}$ = 0.4 mg/mL = *400 micrograms/mL.*
45. 5 × 0.8 g/day = 4 g/day. 4 g per day for 7 days = *28 g.*
46. 1.5 L = 1500 mL; 1500 mL ÷ 10 hr = 150 mL/hr.
    150 mL/hr ÷ 60 min/hr = 2.5 mL/min; 2.5 × 20 = *50 dpm.*
47. 150 mg per 24 hours. $^{150}/_{24}$ = $^{75}/_{12}$ = $^{25}/_{4}$ = $6^{1}/_{4}$ = *6.25 mg/hr.*
48. 28 + 22 = 50 units/day. Stock is 100 units/mL × 10 mL = 1000 units. 1000 ÷ 50 = *20 days supply.*
49. 60 dpm ÷ 20 = 3 mL/min; 3 mL/min × 60 min = 180 mL/hr.
    180 mL/hr × 12 hr = 2160 mL = *2.16 L.* (Check: 180 × 12 = 180 × 10 + 180 × 2 = 1800 + 360 = 2160.)
50. Dose prescribed = 1 mg; dose per measure = 1 g = 1000 mg.
    $^{1}/_{1000}$ × 10 000 = *10 mL.* (Check: 1g/10 000 mL = 1000 mg/ 10 000 mL = 1 mg/10 mL.)

Answers to mock test 2

See also the expanded answers which follow.
1. 300 mg
2. 650 mg
3. 1.5 mg
4. 1 g
5. 3125 micrograms
6. 1 mg
7. 30 mL
8. 2 ampoules
9. 2 mg/mL
10. 5 days
11. 5 micrograms/min
12. 6 tablets
13. 2130 hours
14. 16 mL
15. 42 mL
16. 16⅔ mL/min
17. 80 mL/hr
18. 20 mL
19. 1.7 mL
20. 0.35 mL
21. 300 mg
22. 0.18%
23. 12.5 g
24. 100 mg
25. 5 hrs 33 mins
26. 300 mg
27. 216 mg
28. 200 mg
29. 8 hours
30. 1.44 g
31. 3 bags
32. 5 mL

33. 5 mL
34. 8.4 g
35. 25.8 mL
36. 2.5 mg/mL
37. 40 micrograms/mL
38. 20 mg
39. 8 mg/L
40. 1.67 vials
41. 10 mL
42. 12.5 mL
43. 100 mg/mL
44. 2 mg
45. 50 drops/min
46. 12 doses
47. 125 mg
48. 4.2 mg/hr
49. 15 days
50. 30 mL/hr

Mock test 2 expanded answers

1. 1.2 g = 1200 mg; 1200 mg ÷ 4 = *300 mg*.
2. 50 + 100 + 200 + 300 = *650 mg*.
3. 0.0015 g = 0.0015 × 1000 mg = *1.5 mg*.
4. 250 mg × 4 = *1 g*.
5. 3.125 mg × 1000 mcg/mg = *3125 micrograms*.
6. 500 micrograms × 2 = *1 mg*.
7. Dose prescribed = 90 mg; dose per measure = 15 mg. $^{90}/_{15}$ × 5 mL = 6 × 5 mL = *30 mL*.
8. Dose prescribed = 200 mg; dose per measure = 20 mg. $^{200}/_{20}$ × 1 mL = 10 mL = *2 ampoules*.
9. 20 mg per 10 mL = $^{20}/_{10}$ = *2 mg/mL*.
10. $^{300}/_{50}$ × 5 = 30 mL; 150 mL ÷ 30 mL/day = *5 days supply*.
11. $^{7.2 \times 1000}/_{24 \times 60}$ = $^{72 \times 10}/_{24 \times 6}$ = 3 × $^{10}/_{6}$ = *5 microgram/min*.
12. $^{16}/_{8}$ × 3 = 2 × 3 = *6 tablets*.

13. 1.5 L $= 1500$ mL; $^{1500\,mL}/_{120\,mL/hr} = {}^{150}/_{12} = {}^{50}/_4 = {}^{25}/_2 = 12.5$ hr.
    Finishes at $0900 + 1230 = 2130\ hours$.

14. Dose prescribed $= 400$ mg; dose per measure $= 500$ mg. $^{400}/_{500} \times$
    20 mL $= {}^{4}/_5 \times 20 = 4 \times 4 = 16\ mL$.

15. 12 hours $= 12 \times 60$ minutes $= 720$ minutes. $^{30}/_{270} \times 1000 =$
    $^{3}/_{27} \times 1000 = {}^{1}/_{24} \times 1000 = {}^{100}/_{24} = {}^{500}/_{12} = {}^{250}/_6 = {}^{125}/_3 = 41.667$
    $= 42\ mL$ to the nearest mL.
    Alternative method: 1 L over 12 hours $= {}^{1000}/_{12}$ mL/hr. We
    have 30 minutes $= {}^{1}/_2$ hr; $^{1}/_2 \times {}^{1000}/_{12} = {}^{500}/_{12}$, etc.

16. $^{250}/_{12} = {}^{50}/_3 = 16\,{}^{2}/_3$ mL/min.

17. 120 mL in 1.5 hours $= {}^{120}/_{1.5} = 80$ mL/hr. Check: $80 \times 1.5 =$
    120.
    Alternative method: $120 \times {}^{60}/_{90} = 120 \times {}^{2}/_3 = 80$ mL/hr.

18. Dose prescribed $= 500$ mg; dose per measure $= 125$ mg. $^{500}/_{125}$
    $\times 5$ mL $= 4 \times 5$ mL $= 20\ mL$.

19. Dose prescribed $= 20$ mg; dose per measure $= 30$ mg. $^{20}/_{30} \times$
    5 mL $= {}^{2}/_3 \times 5$ mL $= {}^{10}/_3 = 3.33$.
    Not used $= 5$ mL stock $- 3.3$ mL
    dose $= 1.7\ mL$.

20. 'Dose' $= 35$ Units; 'dose per measure' $- 100$ Units. $^{35}/_{100} \times 1 -$
    $0.35\ mL$.

21. 2% w/v $= 2$ g/100 g. 15 g $\times {}^{2}/_{100} = {}^{30}/_{100} = 0.3$ g $= 300\ mg$.

22. $0.9\% \div 5 = 0.18\%$; alternative: $0.9\% \times {}^{1}/_5 = 0.18\%$.

23. 50% w/v $= 50$ g/100 mL. 50 g $\times {}^{25\,mL}/_{100\,mL} = {}^{25}/_2 = 12.5\ g$.
    Alternative method: 50 g/100 mL $= 0.5$ g/mL; 0.5 g/mL $\times$
    25 mL $= 12.5\ g$.

24. 5 mg/kg $\times 60$ kg $= 300$ mg daily in divided doses every 8 hours
    $= 3$ doses of $100\ mg$.

25. 60 drops per minute $= 3$ mL/minute. 1 L $= 1000$ mL.
    $^{100}/_3 = 333.33$ minutes $= 5$ hours and 33 minutes
    (to the nearest minute).

26. 30 mg/mL $\times 10$ mL $= 300\ mg$.

27. $5 \times 72 \times 10 \times {}^{60}/_{1000} = 5 \times 72 \times {}^{6}/_{10} = 30 \times {}^{72}/_{10} = 3 \times 72 = 216\ mg$.

28. 450 mg $- 250$ mg $= 200\ mg$.

29. 5 mg $= 5000$ micrograms at a rate of 10 mcg/hr. $^{5000}/_{10} =$
    500 minutes $= {}^{500}/_{60}$ hours $= {}^{50}/_6$ hr $= 8\,{}^{1}/_3$ hr $= 8\ hr$ to the
    nearest hour.

30. $20 \times 50 \times 60 \times {}^{24}/_{1000} = 2 \times 5 \times 6 \times 24 = 10 \times 6 \times 24 = 6 \times 240$
= 1440 mg = *1.44 g*.

31. Dose prescribed = 500 mg/8 hours = 1.5 g/day. We have
5 mg/mL in 100 mL bags so dose per bag = 5 mg × 100 =
500 mg = 0.5 g. 1.5 g ÷ 0.5 g = *3 bags* per day.

32. Dose prescribed = 20 mg; dose per measure = 4 mg. ${}^{20}/_4$ ×
1 mL = 5 × 1 mL = *5 mL*.

33. Dose prescribed = 500 mg; dose per measure = 100 mg.
${}^{500}/_{100}$ × 1 mL = 5 × 1 mL = *5 mL*.

34. 400 mg three times per day for 1 week. 400 mg × 3/day =
1.2 g/day; 1.2 g/day × 7 days = *8.4 g*.

35. Dose prescribed = 150 × 86 micrograms. Dose per measure =
500 micrograms. $150 \times {}^{86}/_{500} = 15 \times {}^{86}/_{50} = 3 \times {}^{86}/_{10} =$
25.8 mL.

36. 0.25% w/v = 0.25 g/100 mL = 250 mg/100 mL =
2.5 mg/mL.

37. $20 \times {}^{1000}/_{500} = 20 \times 2 = $ *40 micrograms/mL*.

38. ${}^{4}/_{24} \times 120 = {}^{1}/_{6} \times 120 = {}^{120}/_{6} = $ *20 mg*.
Alternative method: 120 mg/24 hr = ${}^{120}/_{24} = {}^{60}/_{12} = 5$ mg/hr;
5 mg/hr × 4 hr = *20 mg*.

39. 500 mcg/mL × 2 × 4 mL = 4000 micrograms = 4 mg.
4 mg/500 mL = 8 mg/1000 mL = *8 mg/L*.

40. Dose prescribed = 1 g = 1000 mg. Dose per measure = 600 mg.
${}^{1000}/_{600}$ vials = ${}^{10}/_6 = {}^{5}/_3 = 1{}^{2}/_3 = $ *1.67 vials* to two decimal places.

41. Dose prescribed = 500 mg. Dose per measure = 5 g = 5000 mg.
${}^{500}/_{5000} \times 100 = {}^{1}/_{10} \times 100 = $ *10 mL*. (Check: 500 mg is one-
tenth of 5 g. One-tenth of 100 mL = 10 mL.)

42. Dose prescribed = 500 mg. Dose per measure = 4g = 4000 mg.
${}^{500}/_{4000} \times 100 = {}^{5}/_{40} \times 100 = {}^{50}/_4 = $ *12.5 mL*.

43. 750 mg ÷ 7.5 mL = ${}^{7500}/_{75}$ mg/mL = *100 mg/mL*.

44. ${}^{0.05\,mL}/_{15\,mL} \times 600 = 5 \times {}^{6}/_{15} = {}^{6}/_3 = $ *2 mg*.
Alternative method: 600 mg per 15 mL = ${}^{600}/_{15} = 40$ mg/mL;
we have 0.05 mL: 0.05 mL × 40 mg/mL = *2 mg*.

45. 600 mL/4 hr = 150 mL/hr = ${}^{150}/_{60}$ mL/min = ${}^{15}/_6 = $
2.5 mL/min; 2.5 mL/min × 20 drops per minute (dpm) =
25 × 2 = *50 dpm*.

46. 50 micrograms/mL × 60 mL/bottle = 50 × 60 mcg/bottle.
Doses are 250 mcg each: = 50 × $^{60}/_{250}$ doses/bottle = 1 × $^{60}/_5$ =
12 doses per bottle.

47. $^{2.5}/_{10}$ × 500 = 2.5 × 50 = 25 × 5 = *125 mg.*
Alternative method: 500 mg per 10 mL of solution: $^{500}/_{10}$ =
50 mg/mL and we have 2.5 mL; 2.5 × 50 = *125 mg.*

48. 100 mg per 24 hours: $^{100}/_{24}$ = $^{50}/_{12}$ = $^{25}/_6$ = 4.166 = *4.2 mg/hr*
to one decimal place.

49. 100 units/mL × 3 mL × 2 pens = 600 units. 20 units twice
daily = 40 units/day. $^{600}/_{40}$ = $^{60}/_4$ = *15 days supply.*

50. 1 mg/minute = 60 mg/hour. 1g lignocaine/500 mL =
1000 mg/500 mL = 2 mg/mL. Take a 1 hour period to
simplify the working out, then dose in this time = 60 mg and
volume in this time = 60 mg ÷ 2 mg/mL = 30 mL. So
infusion rate = 30 mL in 1 hour = *30 mL/hr.*

Answers to mock test 3

See also the expanded answers which follow.

1. 5 days supply
2. 62.5 micrograms
3. 3 tablets
4. 600 mL
5. 4 mL
6. 400 mg
7. 2 mL
8. 90 mg
9. 331.2 mg
10. 10 mL
11. 2.5 mL/minute
12. 0.12 mL
13. 1.2 g
14. 1 hour 40 minutes
15. 3 bottles
16. 5 mg
17. 3 mL

26. 10 mg/hr
27. 0.8 mL
28. 0.4 mL
29. 1200 units/hr
30. 2 mL/hr
31. 4 g
32. 150 mg
33. 10 mg
34. 0.24 g
35. 15 mL
36. 72 mL/hr
37. 120 mL/hr
38. 4 mL/hr
39. 1.44 mg/day
40. 17 drops/minute
41. 500 microgram/mL
42. 8 mg/mL

18. 100 micrograms	43. 1.9 g
19. 6 mL	44. 22 kg
20. 22.5 mL	45. 1.12 g
21. 15 mL	46. 0.8 mL
22. 4.5 g	47. 10 mL
23. 1.8 g	48. 6 mL
24. 30 mmol	49. 4.8 mL
25. 4 graduations	50. 30 mL/hr

Mock test 3 expanded answers

1. First step: calculate the daily dose in millilitres. Dose prescribed = 1 g per day = 1000 mg. Dose per measure = 250 mg. $^{100}/_{250} \times 5$ mL = 4×5 mL = 20 mL per day.
   Second step: calculate how long the 100 mL bottle will last: 100 mL ÷ 20 mL/day = *5 days supply.*

2. 0.0625×1000 = *62.5 micrograms.*

3. 1.2 g ÷ 2 doses = 0.6 g = 600 mg/dose. Tablets are 200 mg each; 600 mg ÷ 200 mg/tablet = *3 tablets.*

4. First step: work out the volume of one dose. Dose prescribed = 20 mg; dose per measure = 10 mg. Volume = $^{20}/_{10} \times 5$ mL = 2×5 mL = 10 mL per dose.
   Second step: calculate the volume of one bottle. One bottle contains 30 doses = 30×10 mL = 300 mL. So two full bottles contain *600 mL.*

5. 20 mg/kg × 16 kg = 320 mg in two divided doses = 160 mg/dose. Stock is 200 mg/5 mL. Dose prescribed = 160 mg; dose per measure = 200 mg. $^{160}/_{200} \times 5$ mL = $^{16}/_{20} \times 5$ mL = $^{4}/_{5} \times 5$ mL = *4 mL.*

6. 2 mg/mL × 200 mL = *400 mg.*

7. 3% w/v = 3 g/100 mL = 3000 mg/100 mL = 30 mg/mL.
   For a dose of 60 mg: 60 mg ÷ 30 mg/mL = *2ml.*

8. 15 mL × $^{30\,mg}/_{5\,mL}$ = 3×30 mg = *90 mg.*
   Alternative method: 30 mg/5 mL = 6 mg/mL and we have 15 mL; 15×6 = *90 mg.*

9. 5 micrograms/kg/minute for 12 hours = $^{5 \times 92 \times 12 \times 60}/_{1000}$ mg = $^{460 \times 720}/_{1000}$ mg = $^{46 \times 72}/_{10}$ = 3312 ÷ 10 = *331.2 mg*.

10. 2% = 2 g/100 mL = 2000 mg/100 mL = 20 mg/mL. Max dose of 200 mg ÷ 20 mg/mL = *10 mL*.

11. Dose prescribed = 300 mg; dose per measure = 30 mg $^{300}/_{30}$ × 1 mL = 10 × 1 mL = 10 mL (full syringe). Given over 4 minutes = *2.5 mL/minute*.

12. 12 units of 100 units/mL strength: $^{12}/_{100}$ × 1 mL = *0.12 mL*.

13. Concentration of Tegretol = 100 mg/5 mL = 20 mg/mL. One 20 mL dose contains 20 mL × 20 mg/mL = 400 mg. tds = 3 doses per day = 3 × 400 mg = *1.2 g daily*.

14. 1000 mcg ÷ 10 mcg/min = 100 min = *1hr 40 min*.

15. 75 mL/hr × 20 hrs= 1500 mL. 1500 mL ÷ 500 mL/bottle = *3 bottles*.

16. 0.5% means 0.5 g/100 mL = 500 mg/100 mL = *5 mg in 1 mL*.

17. Dose prescribed = 2 mg/kg × 22.5 kg = 45 mg. Dose per measure = 75 mg. $^{45}/_{75}$ × 5 mL = $^{45}/_{15}$ mL = *3 mL*.

18. 1 in 10 000 means 1g/10 000 mL = 1000 mg/10 000 mL = 0.1 mg/mL = *100 micrograms in 1 mL*.

19. Dose prescribed – 300 mg; dose per measure = 500 mg. $^{300}/_{500}$ × 10 mL = *6 mL*.

20. Loading dose = 15 mg × 60 = 900 mg. Maintenance dose = 75 mg tds = 75 × 3 = 225 mg/day. Total = 900 + 225 = 1125 mg. Stock = 50 mg/mL. $^{1125}/_{50}$ × 1 mL = $^{2250}/_{100}$ = *22.5 mL*. (The top and bottom of the fraction have been doubled to give a denominator of 100, which is easier to divide by.)

21. 1.25 mg/hr × 24 hr = 30 mg. $^{30}/_{2}$ × 1 mL = *15 mL*.

22. 0.9% w/v = 0.9 g/100 mL. So a 500 mL pack contains: $^{500}/_{100}$ × 0.9 g = 5 × 0.9 g = *4.5 g*.

23. 0.18% w/v = 0.18 g/100 mL = 1.8 g/1000 mL = *1.8 g*.

24. A 0.18% solution is only one-fifth the concentration of a 0.9% solution: 0.9% ÷ 5 = 0.18% (check: 0.18 × 5 = 0.9). 150 mmol ÷ 5 = *30 mmol*.
    Alternative method: $^{0.18}/_{0.9}$ × 15 mmol = $^{18}/_{90}$ × 150 = $^{1}/_{5}$ × 150 = *30 mmol*.

25. 1.5 mg/kg × 60 kg = 90 mg. Stock is 100 mg/mL × 1 mL = 100mg. Wasted = 100 − 90 = 10 mg. 10 ÷ 2.5 = 4 graduations wasted = *4*.

26. Lock-out time = 6 minutes, which gives a maximum of 10 bolus doses per hour of 1 mL each. Each mL contains 1 mg: 1 mg/dose × 10 doses/hr = *10 mg/hr*.

27. Bolus dose = 20 mcg; dose per measure = 25 mcg.
$^{20}/_{25}$ × 1 mL
= $^4/_5$ × 1 mL = *0.8 mL*.

28. $^{10000}/_{25000}$ × 1 mL = $^{10}/_{25}$ = $^2/_5$ = *0.4 mL*.

29. (5 × 2) + (4 × 1) + 0.4 = 14.4. mL. 14.4 mL × 1000 units/mL = 14 400 units. 24 mL given at a rate of 2 mL/hr: time = 24 mL ÷ 2 mL/hr = 12 hours.
Dose rate = 14 400 units ÷ 12 hours = *1200 units/hr*.

30. Stock = 5 mL × 5000 units/mL = 25 000 units.
Time = 25 000 units ÷ 1000 units/hr = 25 hours.
Infusion rate = 50 mL in 25 hours = *2 mL/hr*.

31. 50 mg/kg × 82 kg = 100 × 41 = 4100 mg = 4.1 g which exceeds the maximum daily dose of 4 g, so *4 g*.

32. 15% = 15 g/100 mL = 0.15 g/mL = 0.15 × 1000 mg/mL = 150 mg/mL; so 1 mL contains *150 mg*.

33. 5 mg tds = 5 mg three times daily = 15 mg/day; 5 mg tdd = 5 mg total daily dose = 5 mg/day. Difference per day = 15 mg − 10 mg = *10 mg*.

34. $^{10}/_5$ × 120 mg = 2 × 120 mg = 240 mg = 0.24 g.
Alternative method: 120 mg/5 mL = $^{120}/_5$ = 24 mg/mL. We have 10 mL: 10 mL × 24 mg/mL = 240 mg = *0.24 g*.

35. 3.054 g = 3054 mg = two doses 1527 mg each. Dose prescribed = 1527 mg; dose per measure = 509 mg. $^{1527}/_{509}$ × 5 mL = 3 × 5 = 15 mL.

36. Stock: 25 mg/mL 10 mL amp; it contains 25 × 10 = 250 mg. 250 mg in 500 mL of infusion fluid = $^{250}/_{500}$ = 0.5 mg/mL.
Rate = 36 mg/hr; take one hour for ease of working out.
Dose = 36 mg; then volume = 36 mg ÷ 0.5 mg/mL = 72 mL in one hour, which is *72 mL/hr*.

37. The pump is on from 2200 to 0700 = 9 hours. The first 4 hours (2200 to 0200 hrs) at 100 mL/hr = 400 mL. This leaves 5 hours for the remaining 600 mL. 600 mL ÷ 5 hours = *120 mL/hr.*

38. 0.1 units/kg/hr × 40 kg = 4 units/hr. We have 50 units/ 50 mL= 1 unit/mL (units/hr = mL/hour) so 4 units/hr = *4 mL/hr.*

39. 1 microgram per minute = $^{1 \times 60 \times 24}/_{1000}$ mg/day = $^{144}/_{100}$ mg/day = *1.44 mg/day.*

40. 500 mL in 10 hours with a 20 drops/mL giving set:
$$^{500 \times 20}/_{10 \times 60}$$
$= {}^{50 \times 2}/_{1 \times 6} = {}^{100}/_{6} = 16^2/_3 = $ *17 dpm.*

41. 0.05% w/v = 0.05 g/100 mL = 50 mg/100 mL = 0.5 mg/mL = *500 micrograms/mL.*

42. Strength = $^{40 \, mg}/_{5 \, mL}$ = *8 mg/mL.*

43. 50 mg/kg × 38 kg = 1900 mg = *1.9 g.*

44. Weight in kg = 2 × (age + 4). For a seven-year-old = 2 × (7 + 4) = 2 × 11 = *22 kg.*

45. 20 mg once daily for 8 weeks: 20 mg × 7 × 8 = 20 mg/day × 56 days = 10 × 112 = 1120 mg = *1.12 g.*

46. Volume of solution = 5 mL. Volume of water added to powder = 4.2. Difference = 5.0 − 4.2 = *0.8 mL* the volume displaced by the powder.

47. 9.7 mL + 0.3 mL = *10 mL.*

48. 9.5 mL + 0.5 mL = 10 mL. Dose prescribed = 300 mg; dose per measure = 500 mg. $^{300}/_{500}$ × 10 mL = $^3/_5$ × 10 mL = 3 × 2 mL = *6 mL.*

49. 5.5 mL + 0.5 mL = 6 mL. Dose prescribed = 600 mg; dose per measure = 750 mg. $^{600}/_{750}$ × 6 mL = $^{60}/_{75}$ × 6 = $^4/_5$ × 6 = $^{24}/_5$ = *4.8 mL.*

50. 10 micrograms/kg/min = 10 × 80 = 800 micrograms/min. Converting to mg = 0.8 mg/min. Stock = 2 × 10 mL × 40 mg/mL = 800 mg. Dividing the stock by the rate of consumption gives the time: 800 mg ÷ 0.8 mg/min = 8000 ÷ 8 = 1000 minutes. 500 mL solution in 1000 minutes = 0.5 mL/min = *30 mL/hr.*